CAPOEIRA 100

Other books by Gerard Taylor

Capoeira Conditioning

Capoeira: The Jogo de Angola from Luanda to Cyberspace

CAPOEIRA
100

An illustrated guide
to the essential movements
and techniques

GERARD TAYLOR

**Photography by Anders Kjaergaard
and Sue Parkhill**

BLUE SNAKE BOOKS
Berkeley, California

Published by Blue Snake Books/Frog, Ltd.

Blue Snake Books/Frog, Ltd. books are distributed by
North Atlantic Books
P.O. Box 12327
Berkeley, California 94712

Cover and book design by Brad Greene

Printed in Singapore

Blue Snake Books' publications are available through most bookstores. For further information, call 800-337-2665 or visit our websites at www.northatlanticbooks.com or www.bluesnakebooks.com.

Substantial discounts on bulk quantities are available to corporations, professional associations, and other organizations. For details and discount information, contact our special sales department.

PLEASE NOTE: The creators and publishers of this book disclaim any liabilities for loss in connection with following any of the practices, exercises, and advice contained herein. To reduce the chance of injury or any other harm, the reader should consult a professional before undertaking this or any other martial arts, movement, meditative arts, health, or exercise program. The instructions and advice printed in this book are not in any way intended as a substitute for medical, mental, or emotional counseling with a licensed physician or healthcare provider.

ISBN-10: 1-58394-176-2 (pbk.)

Library of Congress Cataloging-in-Publication Data

Taylor, Gerard, 1960–
    Capoeira 100 : an illustrated guide to the essential movements and techniques / Gerard Taylor ; photography by Anders Kjaergaard and Sue Parkhill.
        p. cm.
    ISBN-13: 978-1-58394-176-8 (pbk.)
    1. Capoeira (Dance)—Training. 2. Exercise. I. Title. II. Title: Capoeira one hundred.
GV1796.C145T387 2006
793.31981—dc22
                                                        2006024337
                                                        CIP

1 2 3 4 5 6 7 8 9 TWP 12 11 10 09 08 07 06

CAPOEIRA **100** is dedicated to Mestre Sylvia Bazzarelli,
Mestre Marcos dos Santos,
and Professora Agnes Folkestad.

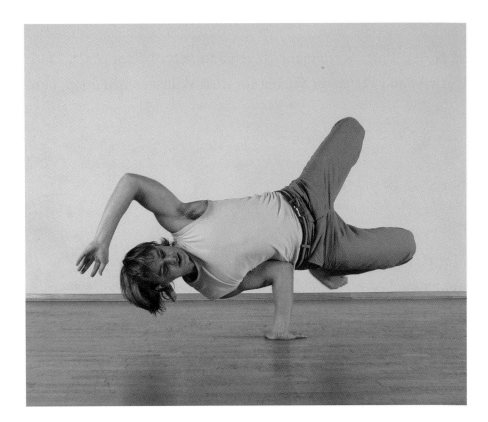

ACKNOWLEDGMENTS

I would like to acknowledge the capoeiristas Tina Kryhlmann (Branca de Neve), Tengil Kryhlmann (Invergado), Ove Nilsen (Axé), Marit Halsvik, and Fernando Sværen for their skilled contribution, hard work, and good humor while doing the movements shown in *Capoeira 100*. Whatever paths we may all take in the future, it will always be a source of personal satisfaction to have played a part in introducing you to the beautiful game of capoeira.

A great debt of gratitude to Professora Agnes Folkestad for being the co-instructor of Oslo Capoeira Klubb, thus making this book possible in the first place. Acknowledgment and warm thanks to Yvonne Cárdenas of North Atlantic Books for coordinating the project from the start, and also to Kathy Glass for the invaluable copyediting of the manuscript. My gratitude also to the team at Blue Snake Books for getting behind *Capoeira 100* with characteristic energy and encouraging enthusiasm.

Tusen takk to Rachel Lewsley for your translation information. Nearly last, though certainly not least, thank you very much indeed to Sue Parkhill and Anders Kjaergaard for going the extra mile to create the great photographs that illustrate the cover and Part One of this book. Also, once again, our gratitude to Rud Videregående Skole for providing the studio.

❖

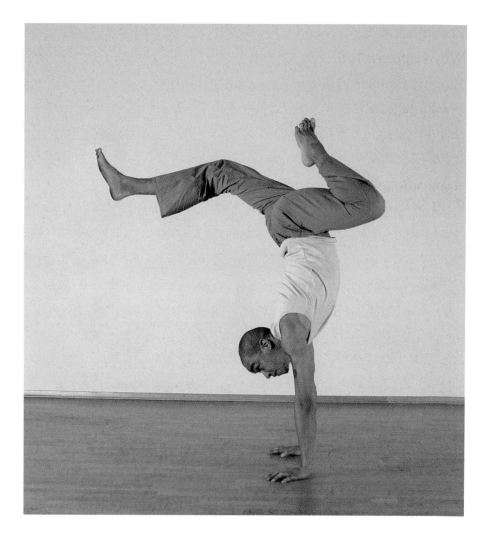

TABLE OF CONTENTS

PART ONE: The Movements 1

Beginner Movements

Intermediate Movements

Advanced Movements

Partner Sequences

PART TWO: The Exercises

100 Capoeira Exercises, Sequences, and Games to improve your skills and conditioning

Please note that the numbers in parentheses under each exercise in Part 2 correspond to the numbers of the specific basic movements involved *as listed and described in Part 1 of this book*. Where alternative movements are possible—as, for example, with different types of aú quebrado or different types of bananeira—the corresponding numbers are depicted with a slash between them. To illustrate, in the Movement section (Part 1), aú normal is No. 16, and two types of cabeçada are Nos. 84 and 87. Thus an exercise sequence in Part 2 involving cabeçada against aú normal would provide reference numbers for more details on the specific moves in the following way: (Nos.16, 84/87). You therefore know that you have a choice of two cabeçadas that you can practice.

Some exercises in Part 2 have (A) or (I) next to the name. This denotes Advanced and Intermediate. The designations mean that these exercises or games include movements from those sections of this book (i.e., the movements in Part 1, separated into Beginner, Intermediate, and Advanced). Or maybe the way the movements are combined in the exercise is better suited for players with some experience. Exercises with no **A** or **I** are suitable for everybody.

Focus Games

Conditioning and Strength Exercises

Advanced Sequences and Conditioning

Miscellaneous Exercises

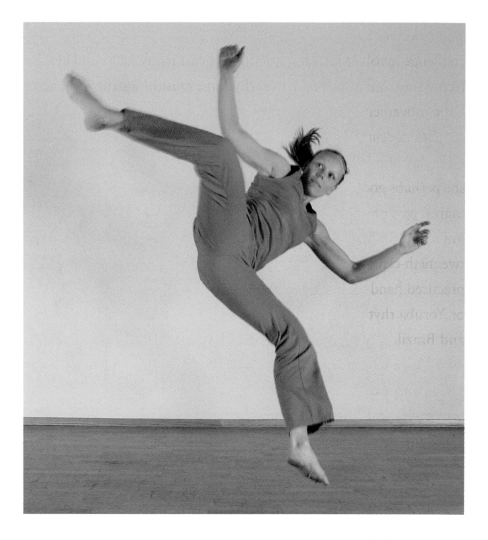

INTRODUCTION

The beginner in capoeira has a challenge and a quest ahead. This challenge involves learning not only a great many kicks and evasive techniques, but also song lyrics, rhythms, musical instruments, acrobatic movements, etiquette, and strategies of play.

The student becomes a historian, a musician, and an athlete almost from day one. The beginner may not realize this, even though he or she perhaps goes home from class having sung about Zumbi dos Palmares, seventeenth-century leader of a *quilombo* (a maroon community in the Brazilian backlands), or Besouro Manganga, an early twentieth-century capoeira outlaw. The *iniciante* (beginner) may have practiced hand-clapping to a time line that comes straight from Bantu or Yoruba rhythms forged by hundreds of years of tradition in Africa and Brazil.

The brand-new capoeira student may have practiced cartwheels, kicks, and exhausting movements low on the ground, which are sometimes confusing and seem to resemble break-dance power moves. To top all this off, they've heard a dozen technique names, all in Portuguese, as well as Portuguese terms for different types of songs and different goings-on in a capoeira *roda*.

Yes, learning capoeira is an inspiring challenge. Notwithstanding the modern "capoeira boom," capoeira isn't fast food. Learning capoeira, staying the course, and truly becoming "formed" as a capoeirista is still the road less traveled, even in Brazil, and even among the people who take classes and begin the quest in this incredible art form.

Why Capoeira 100?

A famous capoeira master named Vicente Ferreira Pastinha once said, "For every strike which is launched there are two defenses already prepared, and for those two defenses, four more strikes. One is [always] improvising and thinking while fighting...."

The way to become a capoeirista is to play capoeira. Not for just an hour or a day or a year, but as a part of your life for many years. To paraphrase another old master, there are not any shortcuts, because there is no end. Maybe there is never a time when one can sit back and say, "Now I know capoeira," because capoeira is like life—there is always more to learn.

When we're young, we have energy and strength, but little experience. We gain experience day by day until we have plenty of it, but then we aren't as young anymore. So every day we adapt and renew our enthusiasm. We develop new strategies to deal with new circumstances. People sometimes say that capoeira is a microcosm of life. It's true, capoeira really is like life, and no matter what anybody may say to the contrary, life cannot be learned from a book.

Therefore, it is first necessary to say what *Capoeira 100* is not. *Capoeira 100* is not a book that is going to teach you capoeira. Learning is an ongoing process that will very likely happen in company with a capoeira group, school, or academy, with luck under the guidance of a capoeira teacher or *mestre* who has already traveled part of the road you're embarking on. Some recommendations for choosing a capoeira teacher and school are given in the question-and-answer section at the end of the book.

What Is Capoeira 100?

Capoeira 100 is a simple guide and reference book for those who are on the capoeira road or are intending to begin the practice. It does not cover every technique in the game of capoeira; it presents representative samples of 100 movements or sequences within the modern *jogo de capoeira*. Each of the techniques or sequence of techniques is accompanied by a photograph or series of photographs to illustrate how they are performed. Text is also provided to describe the technique, how it is achieved, and its possible application within the game of capoeira.

Using the Book

The first section of this book is sub-divided into three parts: beginner, intermediate, and advanced. The moves that are the most easily performed are included in the beginner section. This does not mean that they are less important than intermediate or advanced moves. Many of the basic movements in the beginner section are the most vital in capoeira. Take, for example, the salto mortal and the ginga. Ginga is in the beginner section and salto mortal in the advanced. However, it would be barely possible to play capoeira without ginga, yet completely possible to spend a lifetime in capoeira without doing a single salto mortal. In this context "advanced" simply means that the movement is physically more difficult for the majority of players to perform.

Conditioning

If you have concerns about your fitness to play capoeira and would like to get in shape prior to taking on some of the movements in *Capoeira 100*, a companion volume is recommended for you, titled *Capoeira Conditioning* (Blue Snake Books, 2005). Anybody who can do a basic back bridge, a cartwheel, deep knee squats, and a handstand (the core movements in *Capoeira Conditioning*) will be able to achieve the majority of the movements in *Capoeira 100*. It is important to emphasize at this point that to play capoeira it isn't necessary to perform advanced acrobatics. The game of capoeira can be, and is, played by people of all ages. It's enjoyed by young children and the elderly, by super-fit athletes and people with widely different physical abilities.

Each movement is shown with its Portuguese name. Please note that names differ somewhat according to region or capoeira group in Brazil. So, for example, if you see a movement like aú quebrado and think it looks like bico de papagaio or aú batido, it does. It's the same move called by a different name. The description of how movements are done apply to the capoeira player in the photograph. Not everyone will achieve every movement in exactly the same way. Our bodies are like our fingertips—they appear similar, though each fingertip has a unique set of prints. Likewise, each body is unique to its owner. One player's way of achieving a macaco may not be exactly the same as another's. The guidelines are just that: general directives which you may follow for achieving the technique. If you wish to adapt to your own style or body, that is completely valid. In fact, in some techniques, one or two alternative methods will be suggested.

A Note on Style

Style is considered paramount by some capoeira players. A fair amount of academic energy is spent analyzing whether movement style represents a body memory or *resgate* of capoeira's African-Brazilian past. Some argue that an upright stance and some of the more contemporary techniques of capoeira represent a "Europeanized" or "sportified" version of the "traditional" game.

Capoeira is clearly an art with different "styles" of play. The two most famous forms, which became "codified" during the second half of the twentieth century, are the styles known as Capoeira Angola and Capoeira Regional. *Capoeira 100* takes a deliberate detour around the style issue. When the players pictured in these pages are doing techniques, they are attempting to give the clearest representation of body and limb position, direction of the movement, and so forth. They are in some cases doing static poses, whereas in reality, they would be in motion and also be animated by their own personality and style.

In *Capoeira 100*, where helpful, different choices are supplied for individual techniques—for example, an open or closed aú, or a high or low ginga. In most instances, stylistic considerations are ignored to focus on representing the basic mechanics of the movement and configuration of the limbs.

This is not to underestimate the importance of style in capoeira; it was simply a means to illustrate movements in the most effective way in a photographic format. Some techniques that are strongly associated with Capoeira Regional (e.g. *cintura desperazada*) or Capoeira Angola (various *chamadas*) are not represented, as they are perhaps best learned personally with a capoeira teacher.

Application within the Game

Each movement is accompanied by a suggestion of its applications within the game. Basic principles can sometimes be useful, and beginners will be able to apply these within the roda, especially if you are presently learning on your own, outside a capoeira school or academy. In that case these principles might not be immediately obvious to you. Some basic principles that can be stated in advance are:

1. Always look at your partner. You don't have to look in their eye, you may not even appear to be looking at them at all, but if you are focused properly, you will be concentrating on your partner's movements.

2. Whenever possible try to keep your head between your arms

when doing turning moves like aú, rolé, rabo de arraia, or meia lua de compasso, etc. When your head is between your arms it is better protected.

3. Keep the hands flat when you are doing inverted movements. Try not to do aú or meia lua de compasso, etc., on your fingertips; rather keep the whole palm of your hand on the floor.

4. When you are kicking, aim your foot at your partner even if you are "pulling your punches" (or kicks, as punches aren't common in capoeira). Don't deliberately kick past or away from the other player unless you are playing a game where coordination of simultaneous kicks makes this useful (for example, when two people are doing repeated meia lua de compassos). It is up to the other player to esquiva and deal with your attack techniques as the game dictates.

5. Play close and within kicking range of your partner. Even if you esquiva out of range as a defense, always move back in as part of the game, and don't try to defend yourself by perpetually playing out of range. Try not to play on the other side of the roda from your partner, even if you want room to do acrobatics. Jogo de dentro, the inner game, is always preferable to playing a long way from the other player.

6. Play in rhythm to the music of the berimbau, as it is the music that dictates the game. Do this even if you are playing to a CD.

7. Don't feel you have to be attacking and throwing kicks the whole time during a game of capoeira. Move around the roda and feel out your opponent's capabilities. Capoeira is a defensive game, characterized by the element of surprise. There is little surprise in a machine-gun ratatatatatat of constant attacks.

8. Be aware of legitimate targets for kicks in the jogo de capoeira, which is a different thing from both a streetfight and a full-contact match. Even as a sport, capoeira is not like boxing; you are

not aiming for a knockout. Nor are you in a submission match where you want the other player to tap out. You won't gain points for a hold-down or an ippon for a perfect throw.

Targets are the face, the chest, ribs, and abdomen of the other player. The skill in the game is to keep these areas defended as much as possible. The legs, groin, back, arms, back of the head, and butt are not regular targets for kicks in the game of capoeira, although the legs are targets for foot sweeps and takedowns such as rasteira, vingativa, and tesoura. The back is sometimes legitimate for kicks like aú batendo or aú quebrado.

9. Try to keep your intentions hidden within the game, including hiding an overtly competitive or aggressive attitude, which will inhibit the free-flow of movement between the two players.

10. Generally speaking, it is not good form to do *alto*—high turning kicks such as queixada and armada—over a player who is *already* playing low, near the ground. Flying or leaping over a low-playing partner is acceptable, as are all the low techniques. It is also feasible to kick up, from the ground, at a player who is already in a high alto position.

11. Link two or more movements together in smoothly executed combinations. Kicks, esquivas, and floreios can flow into each other and do not need to be punctuated all the time by ginga. Try not to get into a habit of doing one kick, ginga, one kick, ginga, as this becomes one-dimensional. Link movements imaginatively and train for doing this by working on combinations of movements rather than always on single techniques. Note that there is no contradiction between this advice and the advice in point 7.

12. Use the whole roda for movement. If you stay constantly in the same spot or facing the same direction then you are a sitting target and are not using the space enough. Ginga and aú are

basic movements that are extremely useful for getting around the ring.

·⚬·

Note: To denote the other player, I sometimes choose the word "opponent." The fact of calling another player an "opponent" was convenient and doesn't mean the players are necessarily "opposing" or in antagonistic conflict with each other. It's used here much in the spirit of "opposing" players in a game.

PART ONE

The Movements

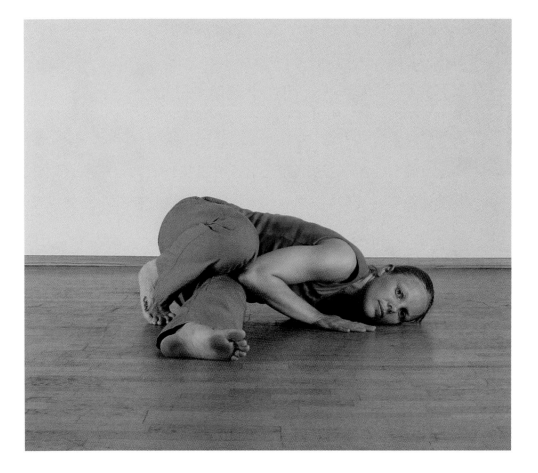

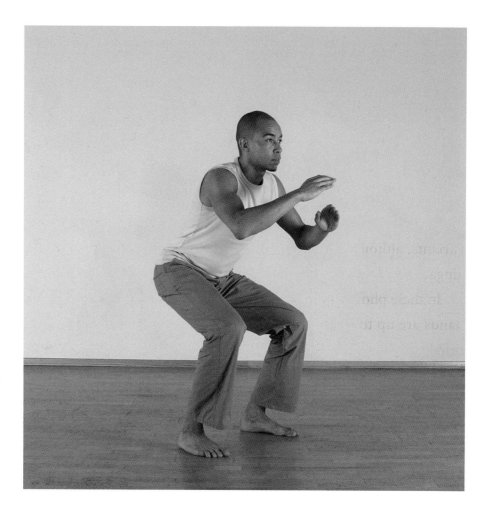

Beginner Movements

1. Ginga

Movement

Ginga is the basic footwork of capoeira. *Gingar* means "to swing" in Portuguese. "Ginga" was also the way that the seventeenth-century Ngola a Kiluanje, Queen Nzinga of Matamba, Angola, spelled her name in written correspondence with the Portuguese.

The movement itself varies. Descriptions given here are basic variants, although each individual has his or her own way of doing ginga.

In these photos, ginga begins in the middle position (fig. 1). Both hands are up to the front of the player's body. In fig. 2, the player brings the left leg back and swaps the weight momentarily mainly to the ball of the back left foot. At this point the left arm is up in front of his torso as defense. From here he pushes off the ball of his back foot to middle position again (fig. 3). In fig. 4 he brings the right foot back, resting his weight on the ball of the back right foot. He swaps arms so the right arm is in front.

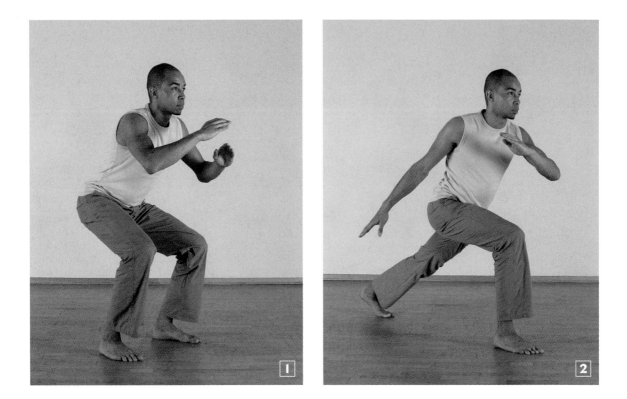

Pointers

Practice doing ginga to music, constantly transferring the weight between your two feet. Try to make the transition of your arm and leg movements well coordinated. The toes of the front foot do not come up when the player puts weight on the back foot, nor does the player actually lean backward with his head and shoulders. Keep both knees bent throughout the ginga cycle and make sure you don't straighten out the front leg at any point. Lower your center of gravity so you feel stable and well-balanced in the ginga.

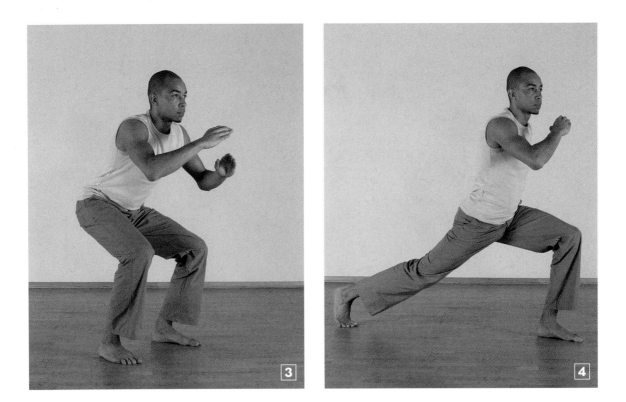

Application within the jogo

Ginga is an important movement and is the cement that holds diverse parts of the game together. Unlike cement, though, the ginga is fluid. The player can ginga whenever they feel like it, as all the techniques bind well together with ginga. The ginga allows the player to keep rhythm; it is a dance step, but it's not a robotic step. In ginga you can move all around the roda, slip under moves, do your kicks and esquivas, and explore the unlimited diversity of movements in capoeira. Ginga can also be used to change direction if you are doing a sequence of turning kicks.

2. Ginga 2

Movement

This illustrates how the same technique can be done in a high or low position. Here the player keeps his arms largely to the fore, his legs are very bent throughout the cycle, his torso sways from left to right, and he stays small and leaning closely over his thighs.

Pointers

Try to vary your ginga to find what suits you best. Experiment with the height, and don't get the idea that the ginga has to be an exact way, with precise hand movements dogmatically adhered to as if they were law. In this case, even when the player is pushing off the back foot, most of his weight is centered over the front foot.

Application in the jogo

If you are playing someone who stays very low and is constantly down near the ground, then it can be useful to lower your ginga so that you are poised to strike at the opponent where he or she is playing. This increases freedom to move unencumbered in the roda, as you are already low and better prepared for the low moves such as cabeçada, rolé, cocorinha, rabo de arraia, negativa lateral, rasteira, etc.

❖

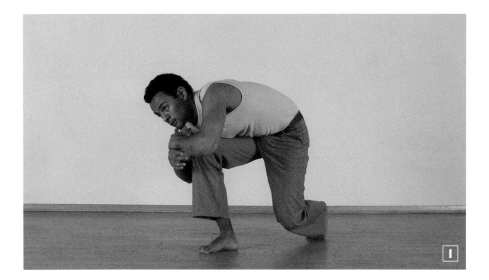

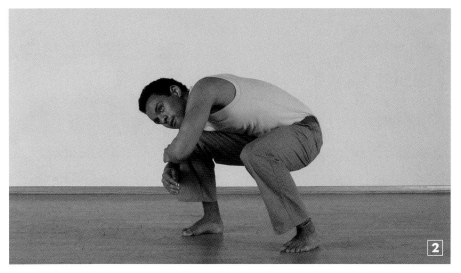

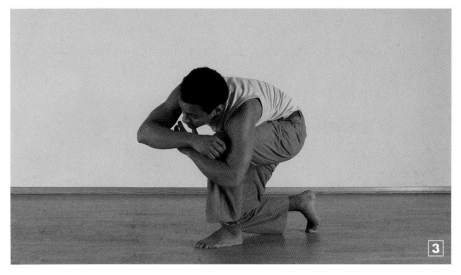

3. Esquiva Lateral

Movement

This is a lateral escape movement, with the weight over the bent leg and the support hand on the floor.

Pointers

Keep the support hand in close to your foot and keep your hips low. Sometimes beginners don't drop the hips low enough and they let their head droop forward, exposing it to kicks. Here you can see that the player's head is protected by her hand. Her body is straight so that the hips are aligned with her legs and spine.

Application in the jogo

This escape technique can slip under turning kicks, and it may be followed up with kicks (such as chapa de costas) or with aú movements or rolé.

✺

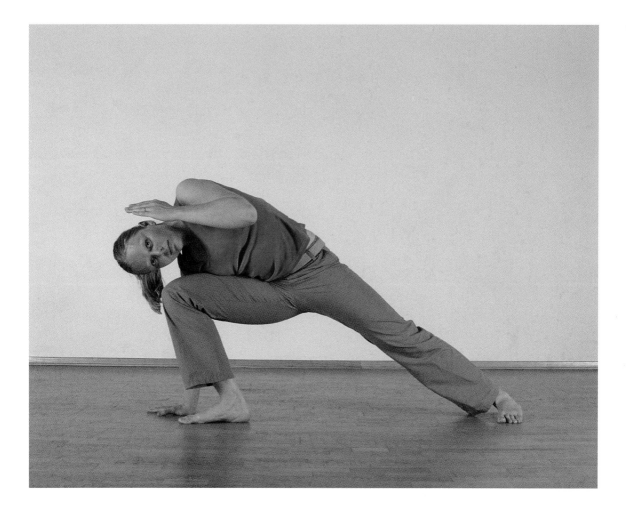

4. Esquiva

Movement

Here there are no hands on the floor. The player leans from the waist directly over the bent leg, making it quick and easy to drop into and come back out of again. The player can drop the torso forward over the leading (front) leg.

Pointers

As your head is still relatively exposed in this esquiva, keep your hand poised defensively for protection of your face. For practice, just ginga and have a partner aim kicks at your head and torso while you use this esquiva to evade them. To change direction quickly, swivel the feet so the toes change direction. At the same time, swing the shoulders, arms, and head forcibly in the other direction, aligned with the toes of your leading foot.

Application in the jogo

At whatever phase of ginga you are in, it is possible to drop very quickly into this esquiva to evade kicks.

✦

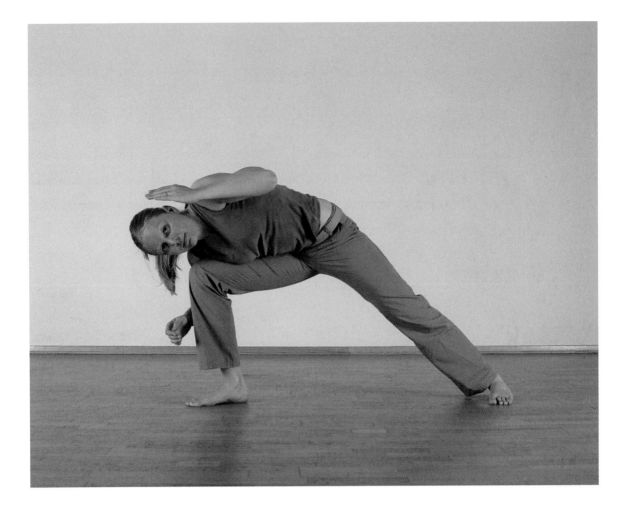

5. Negativa Normal

Movement

In this negativa (shown here from two perspectives), the players have one leg in a squat, the other extended to the front. The support hand is on the floor on the same side as the extended leg. The free hand can protect the face. Some players do this negativa on the ball of their support foot, others on the flat support foot.

Pointers

To get into this position, the player can simply drop into it by bending the rear leg from ginga. Or from ginga, the player can slide the rear leg forward and extend it while dropping into negativa. Practice getting into the position by both methods to give yourself more versatility in the roda. Keep your body weight largely centered over your base foot and support hand. When you drop into negativa or any esquiva that requires a support hand or two on the floor, have your elbows slightly bent to avoid strain on your joints.

Application in the jogo

This popular negativa is quick to fall into. The extended leg is useful for leg sweeps, or it can be thrown up to spin into S-dobrado or chapéu de couro.

✵

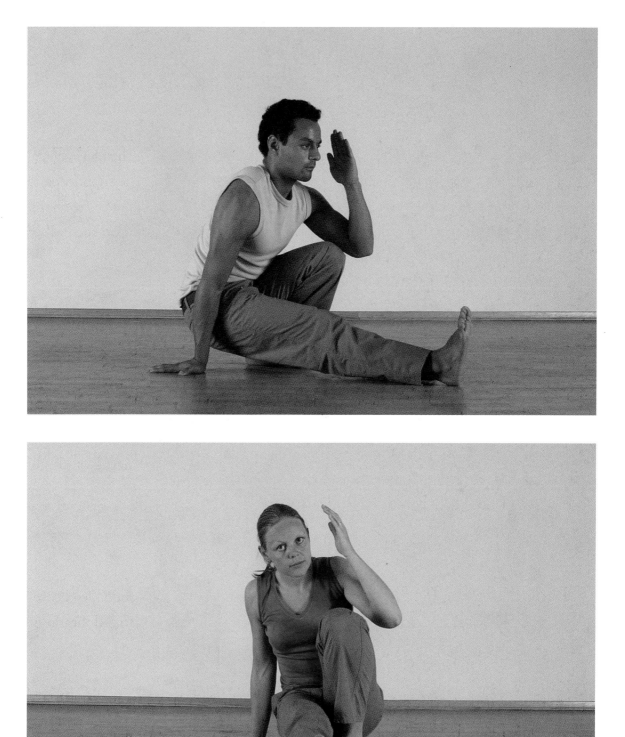

6. Negativa de Solo 1
(NEGATIVA DERRUBANDO)

Movement

Negativa de solo is a negativa on the ground. The inner (left) leg is now extended so that the player can drop as low as possible with the head near the floor.

Pointers

It may look as if the player is lying on the ground, but her weight is held only on her two hands and her feet.

Application in the jogo

This technique is useful, as the outstretched foot can be used for foot sweeps. The negativa de solo can be used in the same way as negativa normal, though it can go lower. The head is already so close to the ground that it is simple to come out of the movement in aú cabeça no chão.

❂

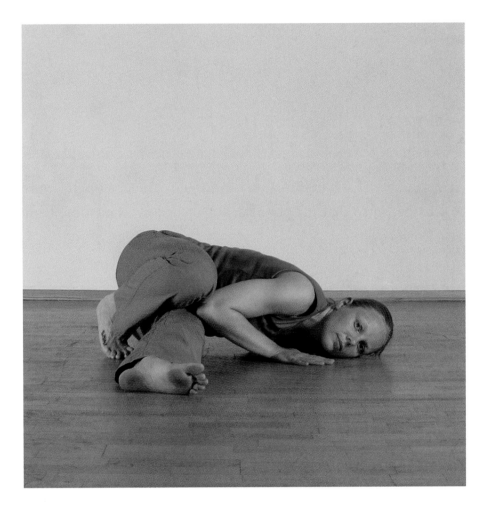

7. Negativa de Solo 2

Movement

This is similar to negativa de solo 1. The difference here is that the outstretched leg lies across the body laterally, while in negativa de solo 1 the leg stretches straight out to the front.

Pointers

Once again, the weight is held on the hands and feet, and the player's body is positioned as low as possible.

Application in the jogo

This is a movement for evading low kicks. It is useful for changing direction while remaining in negativa, simply by crossing over the extended leg from negativa lateral or esquiva lateral to negativa de solo 2. In this way, staying low, the player could, for example, evade rabo de arraia kicks coming from the left and then the right.

✦

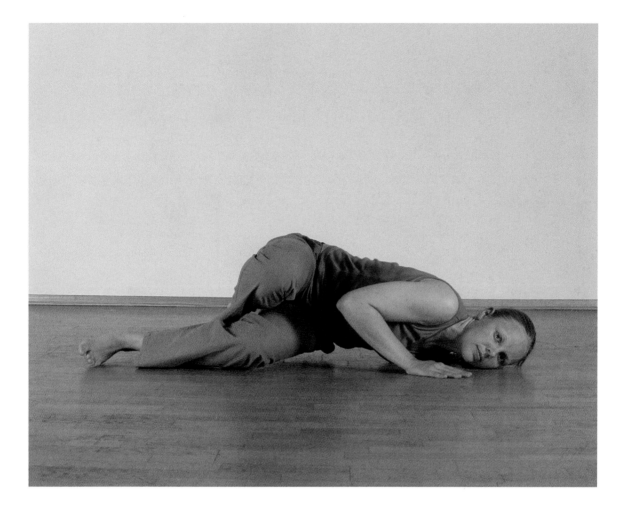

8. Negativa Lateral

Movement

A lateral evasive movement to either side is easily achieved by bending one knee, extending the opposite leg and bending at the waist, and dropping as low as possible.

Pointers

The player's bent (inner left) leg is pointing forward with the knee leading. It is virtually parallel with the ground but doesn't touch the ground. Pointing the knee forward allows the player to go lower without this leg getting in the way of the movement.

Application in the jogo

As with negativa de solo, this technique evades low kicks. It easily converts into low tesoura or queda de quatro—rolé, or aú cabeça no chão. For versatility in the game it is good to be able to play high or low and switch between the two smoothly without weakness in any area. This gives a player the possibility to play with many different types of capoeirista, regardless of their style.

❋

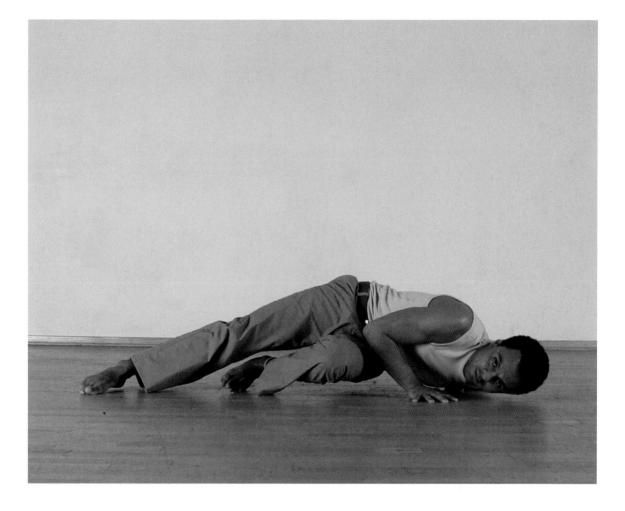

9. Cocorinha
(FIGURE 1)

Movement

Cocorinha actually means "defecation" (thus named due to the squatting position). It is a defensive movement that ducks under kicks. The hands are raised above the head for defense.

Pointers

In this type of cocorinha the player simply drops down very low, with the heels flat on the ground. Concentrate on building up the power and springiness in your legs to move in and out of this esquiva with ease and speed.

Application in the jogo

The player can drop straight down, or step or hop forward into this position under kicks, moving inside strike distance of the other player. The crossed hands, as a last resort, can be raised forcefully to fend off even a front kick such as bênção (although cocorinha isn't the best defense against front kicks). From cocorinha, the player is in a good position to do cabeçada, rasteira, negativa, rolé, aú compasso, negativa lateral or negativa de solo, or even to shoot straight upward for an explosive jumping-turning kick such as armada pulada or a back flip such as gato or macaco.

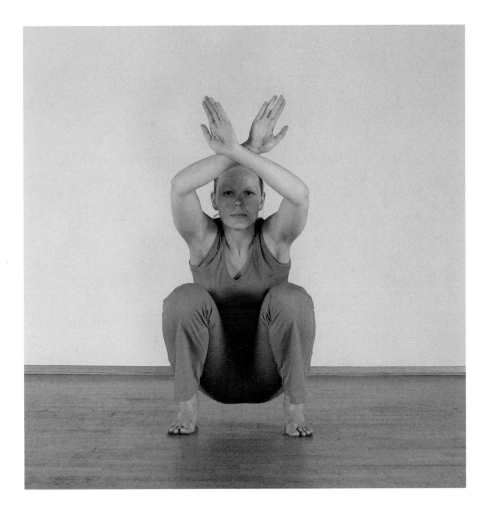

Resistençia
(QUEDA DE COCORINHA) (FIGURE 2)

Movement

This esquiva used to be called queda de cocorinha, though in contemporary capoeira it is more commonly called resistençia. The difference here is that one hand is held on the ground for support.

Pointers

The hand is close to the player's feet, and his weight is on his haunches. If you fall too far back by having the hand too far back from your feet, the position is not so well defended, and you will be slower to spring from the movement.

Application in the jogo

This technique is used as an esquiva to duck under kicks and has similar application to cocorinha.

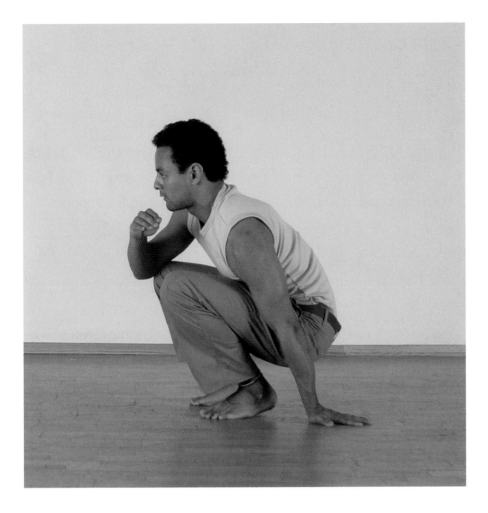

10. Cocorinha 2

Movement

This type of cocorinha has a similar squatting position, though here one or two feet may be raised onto their ball, and the hands closely defend the side of the head.

Pointers

Make yourself small and practice walking backward and forward (like a duck-walk) while keeping the position. In this way you will gain agility to move in and out of your opponent's movements in a low and well-defended posture.

Application in the jogo

This is very quick to drop into from any stage within ginga, without having to readjust the position of your feet. The ability to step seamlessly into or out of cocorinha enables you to move forward and back and change direction quickly without opening up your body. This cocorinha sets you in position to launch cabeçadas and leg sweeps, or to drop further into negativas or rolé.

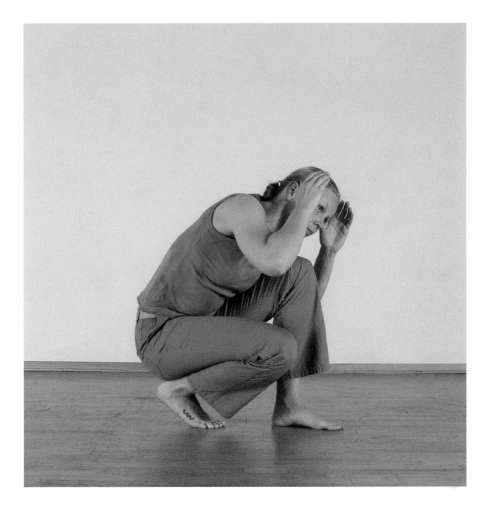

11. Queda de Quatro

Movement

This movement means "falling on four," i.e., two hands and two feet. An early name for it was *movimento de aranha*, meaning literally, "spider movement."

Pointers

Be on flat hands and feet and fully prepared to turn a rolé or a chapa de costas from this movement.

Application in the jogo

This is an esquiva, and also a common transitional stage between other techniques. For instance, a player might drop from an esquiva or negativa lateral, back into a queda de quatro, and then straight into a rolé. Be aware that the queda de quatro is less defended than the resistençia, so don't stay in queda de quatro for any length of time. A player can also walk forward and backward in queda de quatro, which can be useful in a low game of jogo de dentro or jogo de baixo.

❂

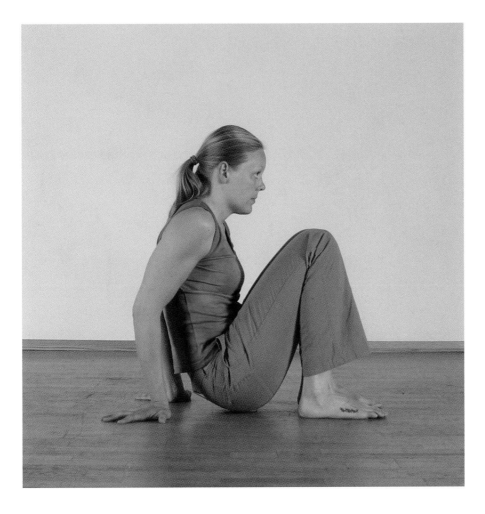

12. Ponte

Movement

The ponte is a back bridge, similar to a gymnastic bridge or back bend.

Pointers

Practice the ponte with your arched back and hips as high as possible, to get a full stretch of your shoulders. The player here has stretched her arms out to full extension and has gone up on her toes for extra height.

Application in the jogo

In capoeira it is not uncommon for players to convert a resistência or even a cabeçada into a ponte to configure their body to see an opponent just by arching their back and reaching over into the bridge. From this position they can drop into a lower bridge or walkover. The ability to ponte well will enhance a player's flexibility and agility in capoeira, where it is the "slippery" player, as much as the muscle-bound, who often takes the advantage.

✳

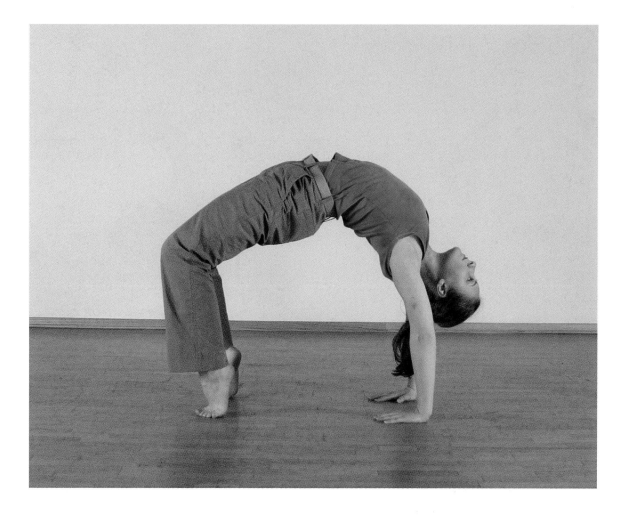

13. Rolé 1

Movement

Rolé means "roll." There are different ways of doing the movement, and in this one, the player is simply crossing one leg around herself, taking it from one side of her body to the other, and to the back.

Pointers

When the player crosses the (left) leg over, she keeps it low, in order to defend her body while doing the rolé (fig. 2). She is looking through the middle of her arms while she does this movement.

Application in the jogo

Rolé is a common movement in capoeira. It helps in moving around the roda while remaining grounded and protected. In the rolé position the player is poised to convert the technique into chapas, rabo de arraia, and aús, to drop into lower esquiva techniques, come up into ginga, or to zig-zag and weave while playing on the floor. It fits hand in glove with movements like negativa and negativa de solo or queda de rins and is used for mobility, defense, and directional changes.

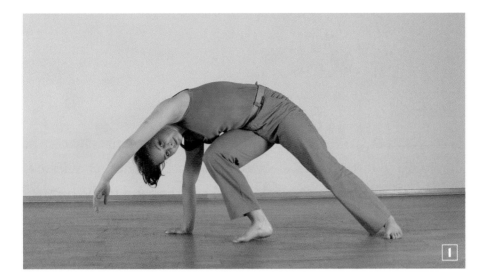

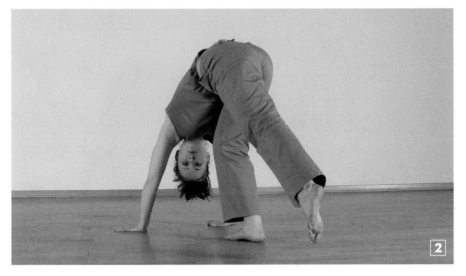

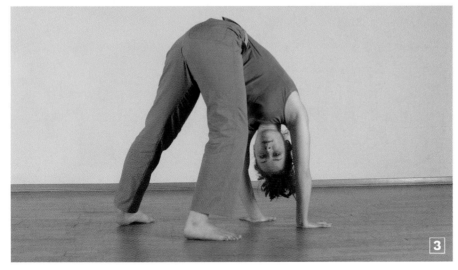

14. Rolé 2

Movement

This is another version of the roll. Here the player simply steps across from one esquiva lateral to another on the other side, always looking through her arms and keeping her hands and feet on the ground.

Pointers

From the fig. 1 position to fig. 2, the player has simply stepped her extended left leg across her body, such that she is now looking through her arms and legs. To complete the rolé, she then steps the right leg around to an esquiva lateral position on the other side. In practice the two steps necessary to get from fig. 1 to fig. 3 should be completed in one unbroken movement. A common mistake is to look over the shoulder while doing rolé, instead of looking through the arms.

Application in the jogo

This rolé has the same applications as No. 13. The main difference is that the player does the whole movement on one lateral line from fig. 1 to 3, as opposed to finishing off by bringing her leg to the back.

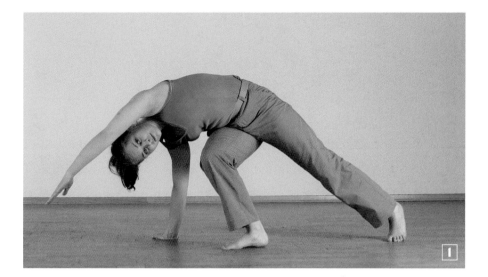

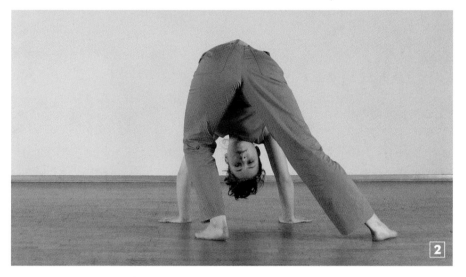

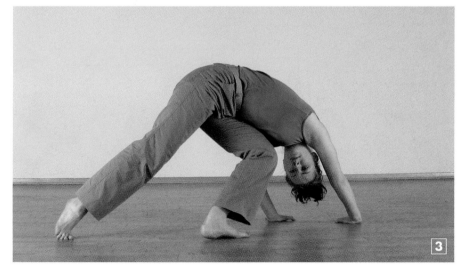

15. Aú Compasso

Movement

This is an aú or cartwheel, though it differs from aú normal in that the legs are kept straight, close together, and aimed downward in front of the player's body. This is a closed aú, defending both the face and torso with the legs during the movement.

Pointers

When you do an aú in capoeira, put the hands straight down toward the floor so as not to telegraph the movement too obviously. Make sure you use the full palm of your hands on the floor for stability in aú, and look in your partner's direction throughout.

Application in the jogo

The aú compasso is a movement for great mobility around the roda, the same as an aú normal, although the player here is less vulnerable to cabeçada and other frontal attacks. It is also easily convertible to aú coisa or chapa de costas. One can turn the aú from an esquiva movement, or following kicks or rolé.

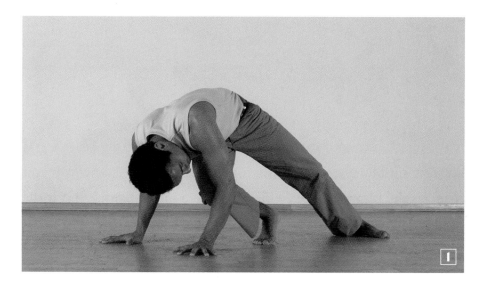

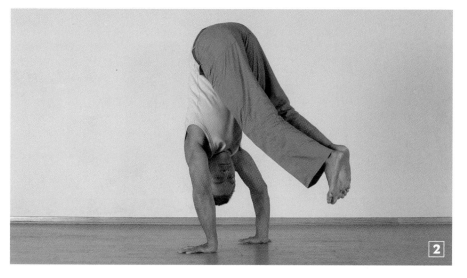

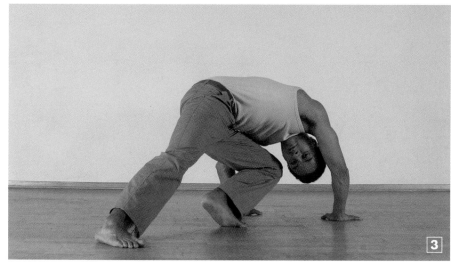

16. Aú Normal

Movement

Aú normal is a cartwheel, and the basis of many acrobatic floreios and attack movements in capoeira.

Pointers

Remember to always look forward through your arms as you do this. Keep your chin in toward your chest so you see upward to the front while you are upside down. Support yourself on the whole palm of your hands. Your feet should be slightly forward to the front of your body as you turn.

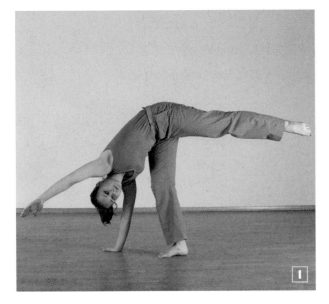

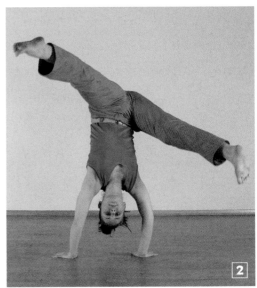

Application in the jogo

Aú normal (or aú compasso) are often used to enter the roda at the beginning of a game. It can be done slowly or at great speed. An agile capoeira player can change directions rapidly with aú, using it effectively to weave around the roda and follow esquivas or to turn under kicks. Kicks can also be converted into an aú—for example, a martelo de estalo wherein the player immediately drops down after the kick and flips over in aú. The reverse is also possible—an aú can be aimed directly at another player and converted into chapa no chão.

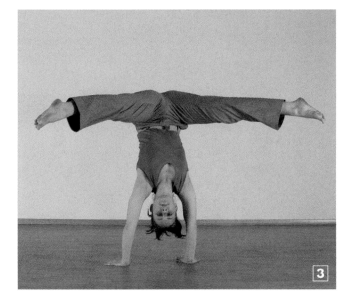

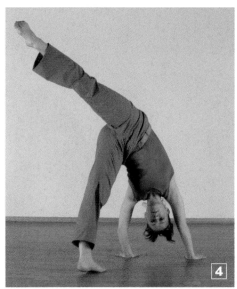

17. Queixada 1

Movement

Queixada means "chin strike." It is a high kick that swings force-fully around the front of the body of the person throwing it.

Pointers

In the pictures, the player is in ginga position with her right leg at the back (fig. 1). In fig. 2, she swings the right leg up and across her body (to the left) in preparation for the kick. In fig. 3, with an all-important rotation of her hips, she swings her leg higher and back in front of her body (to the right), so that the outside of the foot delivers the kick. The foot returns to its original position in fig. 4.

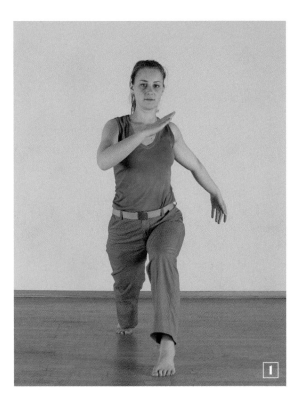

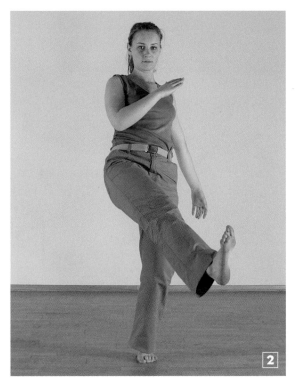

The kicking leg should remain very straight at all points through the kick.

Application in the jogo

Queixada is a very fast kick, and very deceptive. Because the initial phase of the kick swings across the body, then returns back again (between figs. 2 and 3), the other player will oftentimes mistake its eventual trajectory and esquiva off in the wrong direction, making it a useful kick to set them up for a trap. It is also an excellent lead-in for a sequence of kicks such as armada and meia lua de compasso, which can all follow one after the other in a series of spins, without being broken up by ginga.

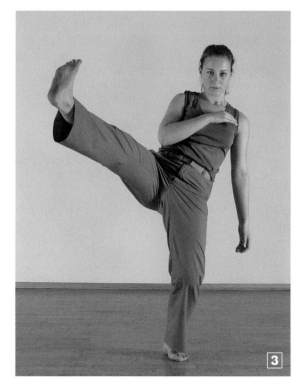

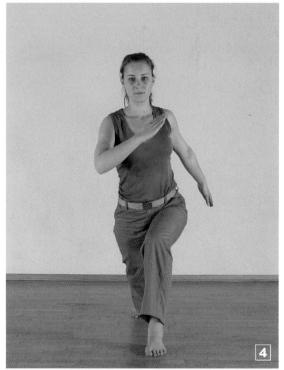

18. Queixada 2

Movement

This is the same as the previous kick, only in this case you kick with the front leg instead of the back leg.

Pointers

In fig. 1 the player's weight is on her front (right) foot. She slides her left foot up behind the right foot (fig. 2). At this point she transfers the weight to the back (left) foot in readiness for the kick. Having transferred the weight fully onto the left foot, she swings the right leg fully across the front of her body, being sure to keep the kicking (right) leg completely straight. She brings it all the way to the back to ginga position (fig. 4).

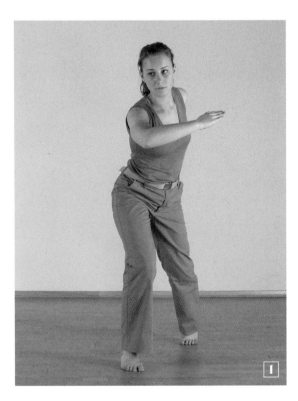
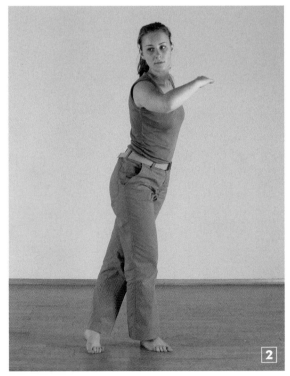

Make sure the swing of the kick makes one smooth arc in front of the body, as if your waist is a fast-turning cylinder, the kicking leg a piece of rope attached to it, with a brick tied to the end of the rope. The "brick" is spun around at great speed by the force created by the cylinder's rotation. Once you reach the kicking point (fig. 3), immediately pull the leg back and down toward the fig. 4 position.

Application in the jogo

The fact that this kick is achieved with the front leg and involves a step-up means that it can be used to move forward toward your partner to close ground in the roda. Switching between queixadas 1 and 2 is confusing for the opponent, and these kicks are also perfect for directional changes at high speed. Note that Capoeira Angola players generally don't use queixada very often.

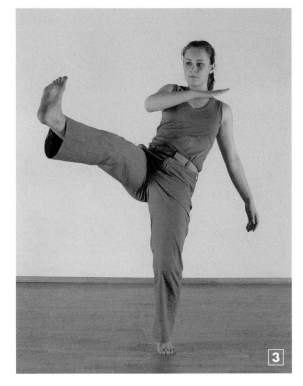

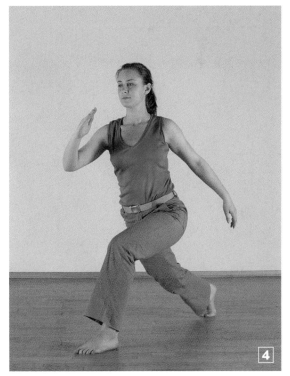

19. Armada

Movement

Armada literally means "armed strike." It is a very fast 360° turning kick delivered with the outside edge of the kicking foot.

Pointers

As you rotate, the correct sequence is to turn your head first, then shoulders, then hips, and finally, when you have spun your whole head, torso, and hips to full stretch, deliver the kick. You are already looking forward (as in the photos) over your shoulder at your target. A common mistake is to try to kick before having turned the head, shoulders, and hips fully in preparation. This leads to kicking backward (away from your target) or incorrectly kicking with the heel of your foot with a bent leg, rather than the outside edge of your foot with toes upward and a straight leg (correct).

The back leg is the kicking leg, and it returns to the same spot where it began. The supporting leg and foot should be securely planted on the ground. Even though you will pivot on the support foot, try not to hop, as this would leave you vulnerable to foot sweeps. Try to drill the support foot into the ground as you pivot on it for the kick. The support leg can be slightly bent when you kick, though the kicking leg should be completely straight.

Application in the jogo

Armada is a popular kick in all styles of capoeira. It can be used in a fast game, and executed repeatedly and quickly. This versatile kick can be delivered at waist or head height and easily linked to a set of turning kicks which might include queixada, meia lua de compasso, or parafuso. Many players step forward immediately prior to the armada, or step back and then throw it. By shifting legs with a step, it makes it more difficult for one's opponent to sense where the kick is coming from, and allows a player to correct the distance for the kick.

✦

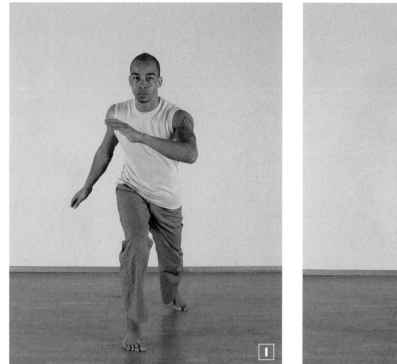

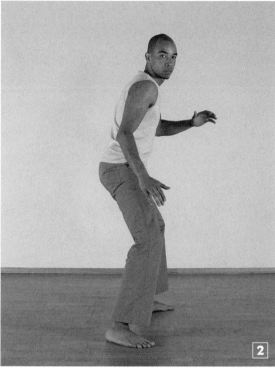

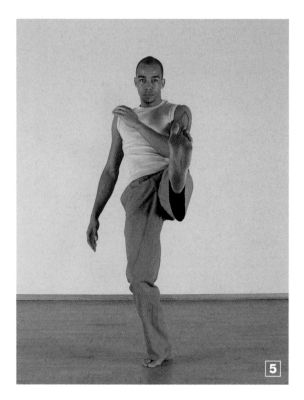

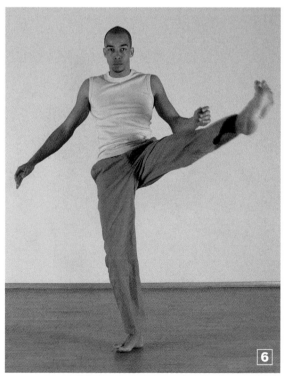

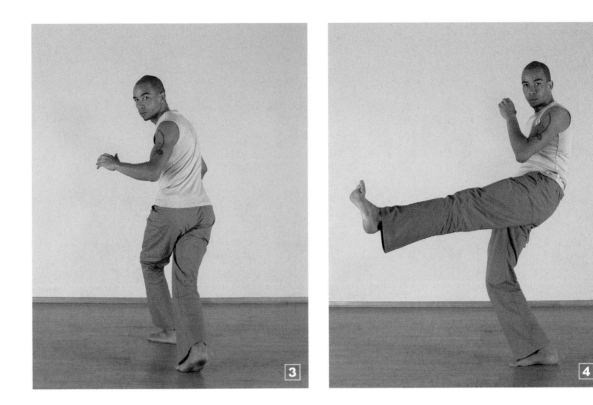

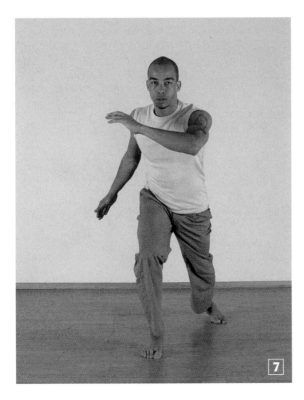

20. Bênção

Movement

This is a front kick with the sole of the foot, sometimes called *chapa de frente*.

Pointers

Bring the knee up before kicking (fig. 2), then push forward powerfully with your hips for leverage as you extend the kicking leg. Pull the toes back, so you kick mainly with the sole at the heel end of your flat foot (fig. 3). Let the arms splay out relaxed to the sides as you kick. The supporting leg can be bent. Keep the whole sole of the support foot on the floor, and try not to come up on the toes.

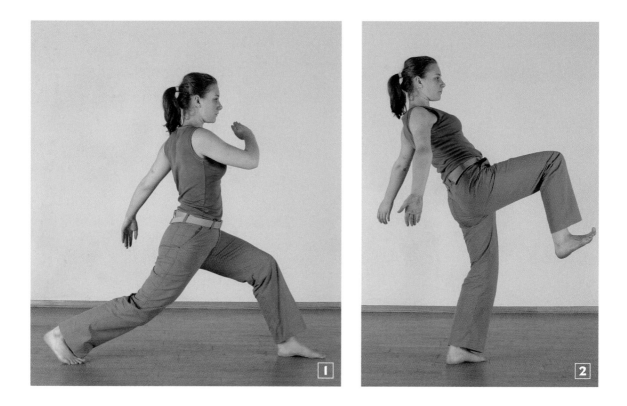

Application in the jogo

This traditional capoeira kick is solid and fast. It can be aimed at head or waist height. As with other fast and direct kicks, don't deliberately aim to the side of your opponent with this kick, but use it to test esquiva skills, which will have to be fast to avoid the bênção.

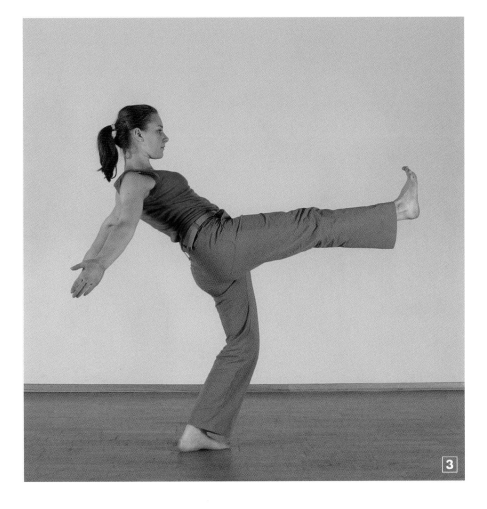

21. Meia Lua de Frente
(MEIA LUA)

Movement

This is sometimes called simply meia lua: a half-moon kick to the front, delivered with a straight leg stretched forward by an extension of the hips

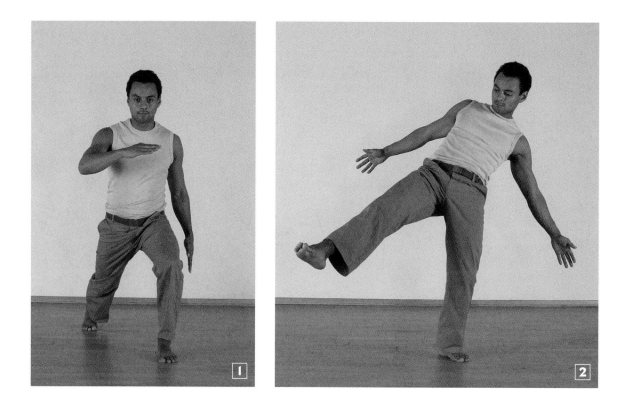

Pointers

Keep the kick low. The kicking leg is straight and the hips are pushed forward as the meia lua sweeps across the front of your body (fig. 2). This kick can be done very slowly or at a medium tempo and is popular in Capoeira Angola. The arms can be splayed out relaxed with open hands. Finish the kick when it reaches a point directly in front of you (fig. 3). Return to ginga without bending the kicking leg too much to get there.

Application in the jogo

This is a good kick to feel out your opponent's style. Because it is low and frontal it doesn't leave you vulnerable to sweeps or counterattacks.

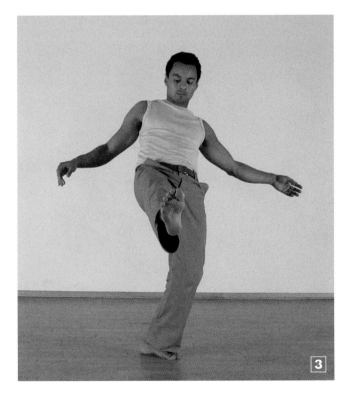

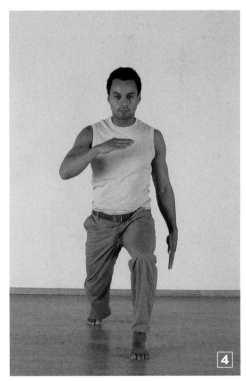

22. Ponteira 1

Movement

This technique is a front kick delivered with the ball of the foot. Here, the back leg simply swings up in a fast arc, as if to kick directly under the chin of the intended target (fig. 2).

Pointers

Keep the support foot flat on the floor and remain well grounded. In this version of the kick, the leg remains straight as it swings up, and thus the trajectory of the kick is mainly upward.

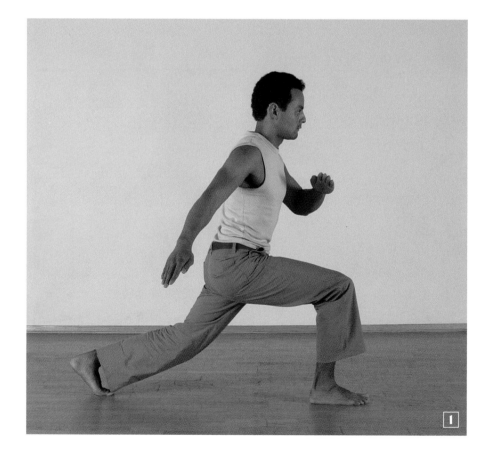

Application in the jogo

A straightforward attacking front kick, the ponteira can be used in a game where the players are in a more upright position, and it should be delivered at speed, being more appropriate for a faster game. It can leave the player throwing it vulnerable to foot-sweep counter-attacks, which is another reason for kicking fast.

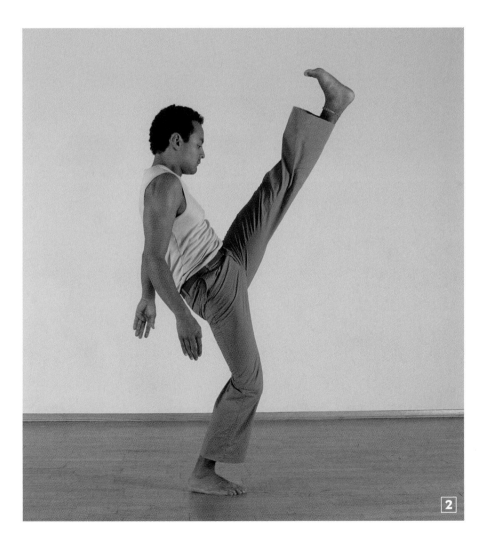

23. Ponteira 2

Movement

Here the ponteira is directed not only upward, but also forward. It differs from bênção because the surface to kick with is the ball of the foot. The back leg is lifted, knee first, and then thrust forward at the belly, solar plexus, or face of the other player (fig. 2).

Pointers

Once again, keep your support foot flat on the floor, and sink your weight down into it as you thrust forward with the hips. This will

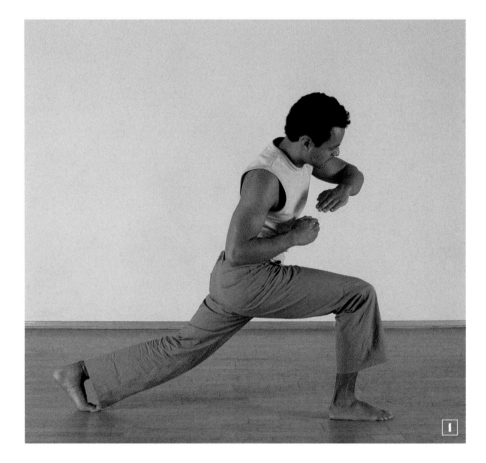

give you more power and leave you less vulnerable to foot sweeps. The arms can come out to the side as in fig. 2. Make sure you are not standing too close to the other player when you do ponteira. Your distancing should be correct, giving room to reach an opponent with the kick, including an added thrust forward from the hips for extra power.

Application in the jogo

Similar applications to bênção and ponteira 1: a front kick to make direct attacks at a higher target.

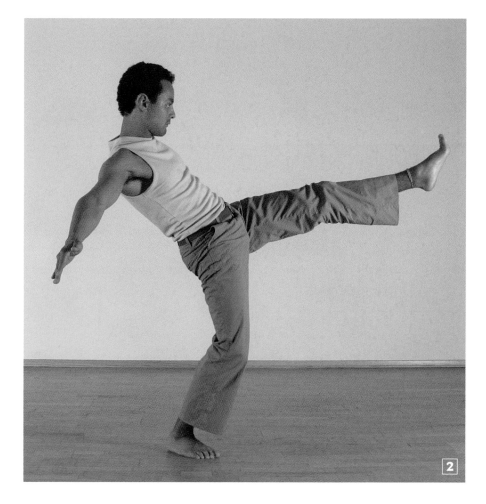

24. Chapa

Movement

This is a side kick. In practice it can be delivered either with the front leg, which requires a sidestep, or as shown in the photographs here, directly with the back leg.

Pointers

In fig. 2, when the player brings his knee up, it is directly in front of his body. This is both protection for him and a perfect starting point for delivery of the chapa. Make sure that your raised knee is directly in front of the center line of your body before you deliver the chapa.

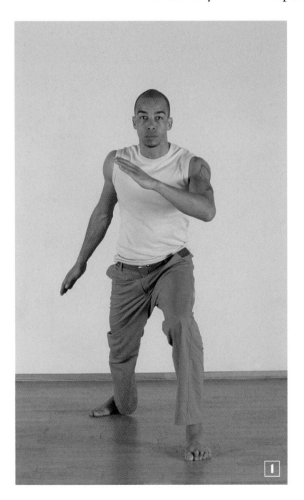

Notice that the player's left (supporting) foot is directed with toes to the front in fig. 1, though in fig. 2 the support foot has swiveled so the toes are directed halfway and then almost to totally to the rear (fig. 3). This swiveling of the support foot allows for a more stable balance, and greater height and ease when kicking. As you kick, look at your target and make sure your hips are forward, giving extra reach and power to the kick.

The flat sole of the foot (particularly the heel-end) is the strike surface for the kick. Be careful when doing fast and powerful kicks into mid-air that you do not snap them out too forcefully, which might damage your knee.

Application in the jogo

This chapa can be delivered with enormous speed and power. This is not a good reason to deliberately miss the target with it (by aiming it in the wrong direction). Instead it is usually preferable to do the kick more slowly or pull it up short of the target, while kicking in the correct direction.

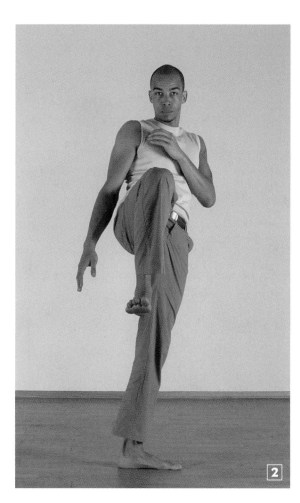

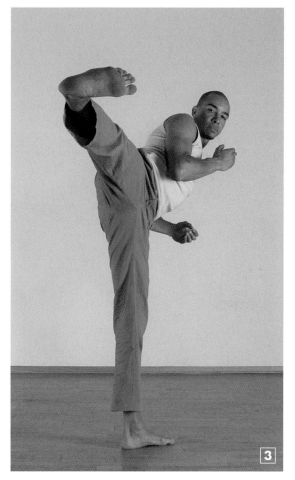

25. Chapa Giratório

Movement

This movement is similar to the chapa, although it is "gyrating," meaning that the player rotates quickly and follows the turn by blasting a powerful chapa from the back leg.

Pointers

In the photographs, the player begins in ginga position. In fig. 1 his left leg is at the back. In fig. 2, he rotates his whole body to the left from the waist, so that he is looking to the front over his left shoulder at his target **before** beginning the kick. Having positioned himself perfectly to begin, the player fires the chapa directly at the target (fig. 3).

When doing chapa giratório, make sure the chapa jabs out to the front of the body and is not delivered as a turning kick in the same way as an armada. The rotation is preliminary to the kick; the kick itself does not turn but drives directly forward at the target in a similar way to chapa. Make sure you have the correct distance for this kick before you do it, because if you are too far from your opponent the kick will miss, and if too close you will get tangled up with him. It is worth practicing this with many repetitions to get a good feel for the length of your legs and where you need to be standing for maximum impact with the kick.

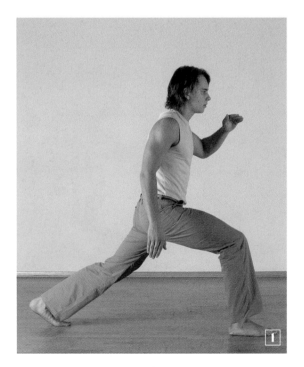

It is also recommended to exhale forcefully into the kick, and sink your weight into your supporting leg and foot to gain stability. Remember that the strength for the thrust of a kick comes equally, if not more, from your supporting leg as from your kicking leg. Sinking your weight into your support leg also leaves you less vulnerable to being swept with a rasteira while kicking.

Application in the jogo

This is a very surprising kick. The rotation of the body can be achieved so swiftly that the kick is virtually delivered before the other player sees it coming; and if they do, as often as not they will mistake it for an armada and prepare to escape with esquiva lateral or attack with a rasteira, in either case walking directly into the kick. In the photos, the chapa giratório is delivered at head height, although it can be lower. Remember always to control kicks so as to avoid injuring the other player, especially if they are inexperienced and liable to esquiva into the kick by mistake.

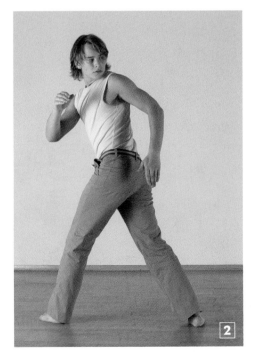

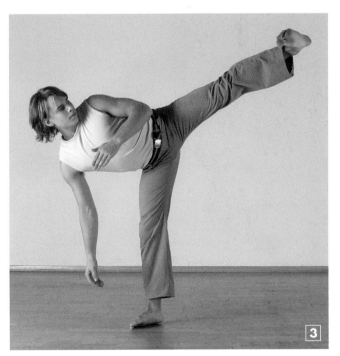

26. Chapa de Costas 1

Movement

This is a straight kick delivered to the back, while looking through the arms and to the inside of your support leg.

Pointers

This kick begins with a bent knee and then jabs straight at the target like a spike. The sole of the foot is the striking surface.

Application in the jogo

This kick is powerful due to its simplicity, speed, and the fact that it has a base of three limbs on the floor rather than one. The triangular pattern of the two support hands and foot make for an ultra-stable foundation from which to strike the target. The kick can be delivered at many points in the game—for example, halfway through a rolé, or immediately as a player falls forward out of a bananeira.

✸

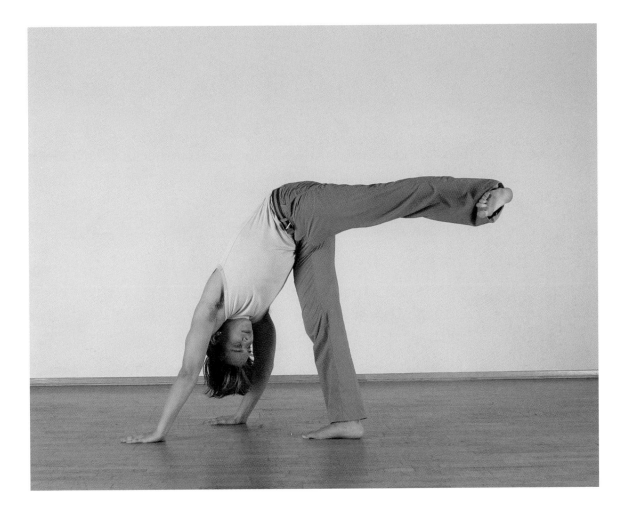

27. Chapa de Costas 2

Movement

This is a straight kick delivered to the back, while looking through the arms and to the outside of your support leg.

Pointers

The same points apply to this kick as to the previous technique. You can see from the photo that the player is looking to the outside of his support leg. In training, try to vary your techniques and practice both types of chapa de costas. Be careful when doing chapa de costas not to kick lazily at any old target, or to kick in mid-air. Kick to the open areas of your opponent's body to create strategic logic in the game.

Application in the jogo

The same applications apply as for the previous technique, with the exception that the player is looking outside his support leg, which may come as a surprise. Remember to begin the kick with a relaxed leg, bent fully at the knee, and then jab out directly at your target.

❂

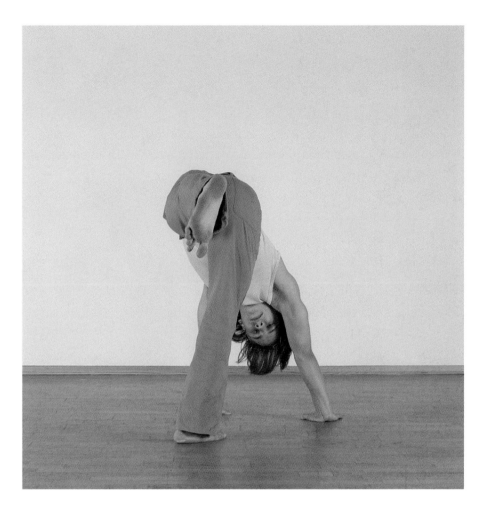

28. Chapa no Chão 1

Movement

This is a chapa side kick. The player sidesteps toward the target and places his rear hand on the floor at the same moment as he kicks.

Pointers

From fig. 1, step behind your front leg quickly to close the gap between you and your partner (fig. 2). Drop the rear hand to the floor and extend the kicking leg to impact at exactly the same moment that your hand hits the floor (fig. 3).

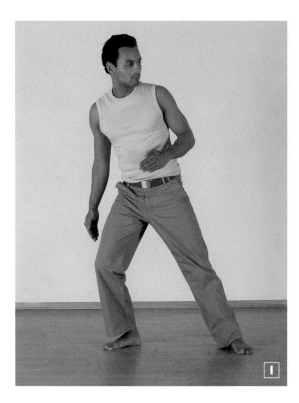

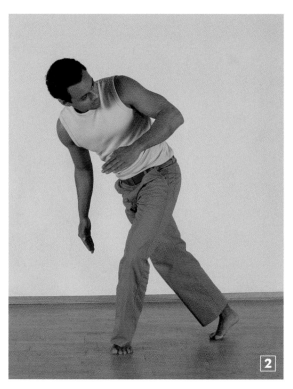

Application in the jogo

This is slightly different from chapa de costas, as you execute the chapa as a side kick, and instead of already being on the floor, your hand will touch down to give added support and balance to the kick at the moment of impact. In this case the side step is a very quick way to move toward the opponent and provide even more momentum to the movement in advance. Due to the hand being on the floor at its conclusion, the kick can be followed up with aú to back away from the opponent, a bananeira, or hand spin.

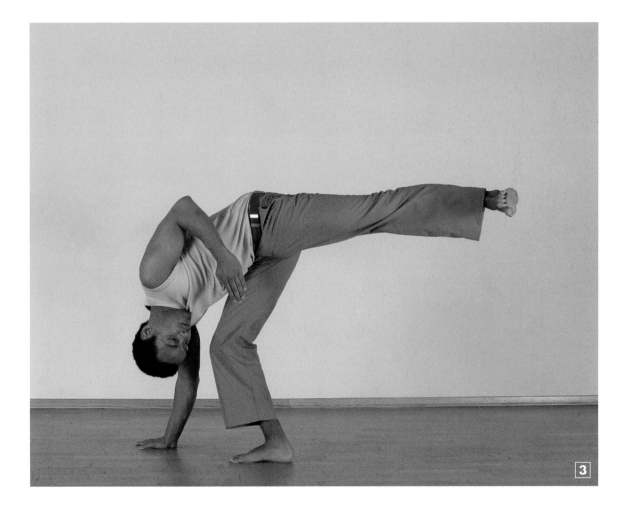

29.

Chapa no Chão 2

Movement

From a queda de quatro position (fig. 1), the player raises her leg and pushes up and forward with her lower back and hips, kicking straight above herself (fig. 2).

Pointers

When you kick, if you want to rise on the toes of the support foot for extra height, it is feasible. Kick with the sole of the foot.

Application in the jogo

As queda de quatro is a potentially vulnerable place to be, this kick is a good "defense attack" against a player to the front, whether he or she is standing or on the ground.

※

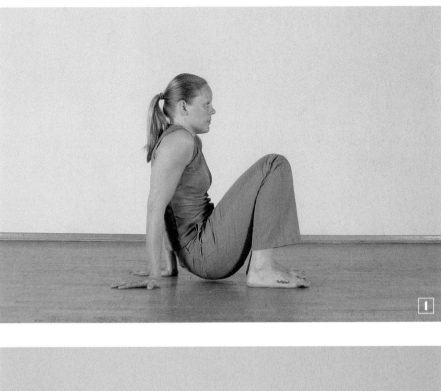

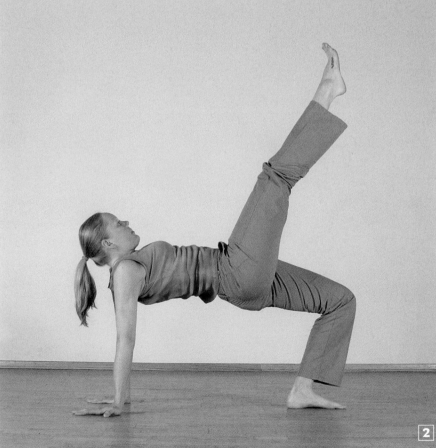

30. Martelo de Estalo

Movement

This is a roundhouse kick delivered straight from the back leg in ginga.

Pointers

As with chapa, bring your knee up in front of your body for positioning and protection (fig. 2). The support foot can swivel back to put it at a better angle to your body to do the kick. When you kick (fig. 3), straighten the leg forcefully, so that the kicking surface is the top of your foot. Despite the name "cracking hammer," if you are not kicking a bag but practicing the kick in mid-air, try not to snap it out too hard or you might create knee problems.

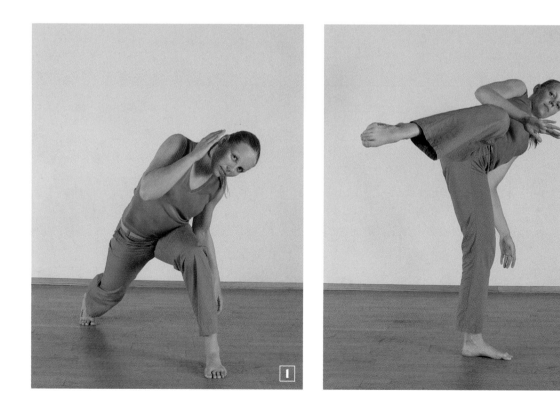

Application in the jogo

Up until the kick is delivered it is difficult for an opponent to tell whether this is a roundhouse kick or a side kick (chapa), so it is useful for surprise, especially in a game characterized by many turning kicks, where a player might get complacent expecting predictability, and this can come out of nowhere, against the tide. It can be aimed at head, shoulder, or rib height.

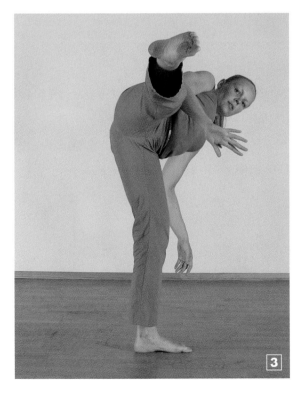

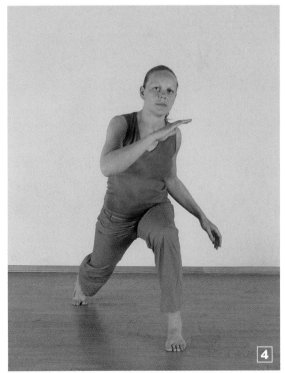

3**1.** Martelo Giratório

Movement

This is a simple but surprising technique that reverses the meia lua de compasso idea of a spinning kick on the hands, so that in this case instead of kicking with the heel first, you kick with the top of the foot.

Pointers

From the fig. 1 position, create a spin by pushing with the hands, straightening the support leg slightly, and rotating the hips. Throw the leg completely around 180° in front of your body so that it comes down the other side. The kicking surface is the top of your foot (see fig. 2). Remember to look through your arms at your target.

Application in the jogo

Do martelo giratório quickly and with power. As a slow movement it can be bland and formless. Interspersed with fast-moving circular kicks it often catches the partner off guard. In fig. 3 at the end of the movement, there are many follow-ups; for example, the player could drop and slide forward his right leg for a negativa de solo and then come up with a chapa no chão. This kick also fits well with turning meia lua de compasso movements, to keep spinning in the same direction though with the other foot.

❖

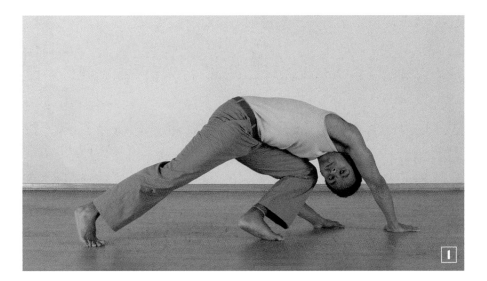

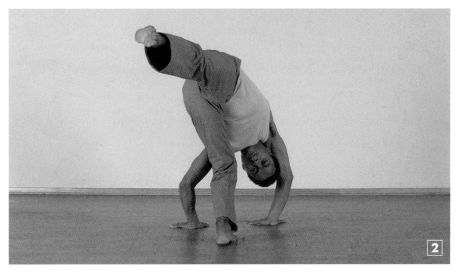

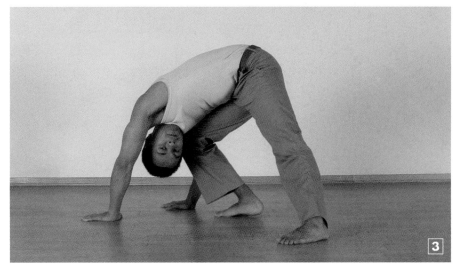

32. Meia Lua de Compasso

Movement

The name of this movement is "Half Moon in a Compass." In the picture the player is kicking with her right leg, and the left foot is the point of the compass around which the kick rotates.

Pointers

Meia lua de compasso can be done with two hands on the floor, looking between your arms at your target, or, as in these photos, with one hand on the floor, the other up in front of the face for protection. In fig. 2, the player bends double and looks at the target **before** beginning the kick. The principle of turning the head and looking at the target before kicking holds true in all turning kicks. The swing down of the head and torso from the ginga position (between figs. 1 and 2) provides enough momentum for the kick itself (fig. 3). Keep the kicking leg very straight (although the support leg can be as bent as you like) and direct the swinging heel of the kicking foot directly at your intended target.

After the kick (the back foot having swung 180° from the start position), the player begins to come back to an upright position again (figs. 4 and 5). Notice that she doesn't at any point bring her head forward in front of her body. Her head goes down to the back during the kick, and then to upright again. Never stick your head forward to the front of your body during the meia lua de compasso. If you are kicking with the right leg, it is the left hand that will go on the floor as you kick. Keep the elbow of the free protecting arm in to your side, and the hand up near your face. Finish by returning to the start position (fig. 6).

Application in the jogo

The meia lua de compasso is a higher version of the traditional rabo de arraia kick. Most kicks in Capoeira Angola are delivered at waist height or below, whereas the meia lua de compasso is high enough to aim at the head of a person standing upright.

Meia lua de compasso can be used in different ways according to the type of game being played. It can be aimed directly at the target areas of the other player's body (face, chest, ribs, belly). It can also be used as part of a close and fast game, in unison and with another player, so they both spin around, coordinating meia luas. Meia lua de compasso is often used in this way for demonstrations.

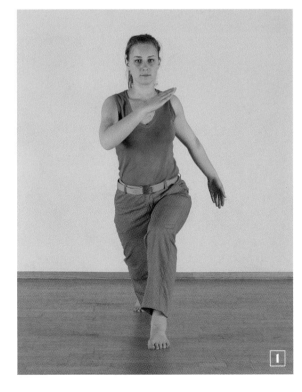
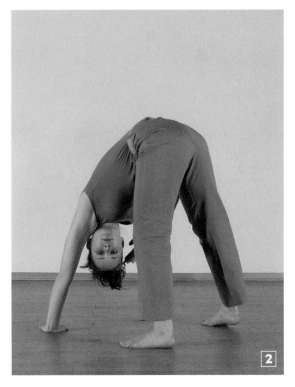

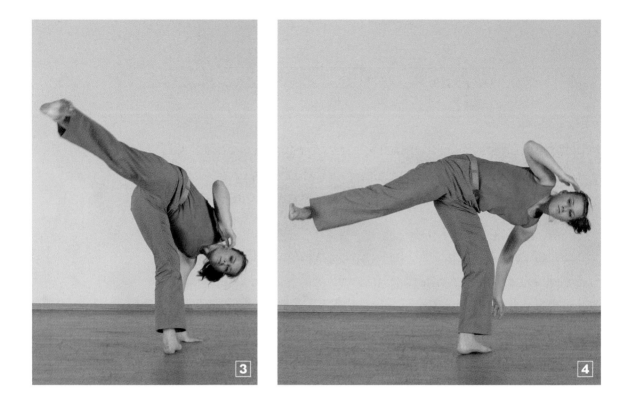

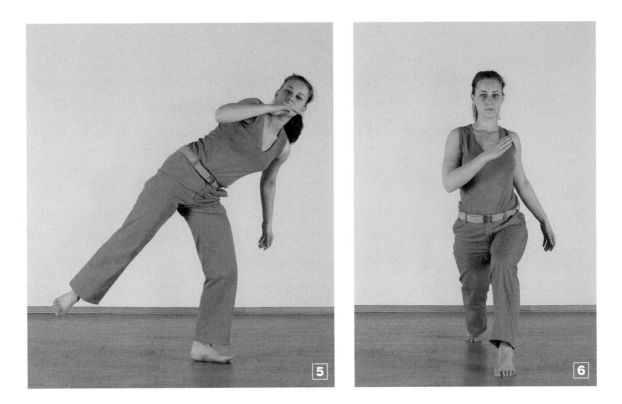

33.

Rabo de Arraia

Movement

This movement is similar in principle to meia lua de compasso, and indeed the term "rabo de arraia" may be used by some people to describe meia lua de compasso. The distinction is made here because the player is executing the kick lower (fig. 3), making it more suitable for a game played low to the ground. To kick low like this is sometimes called *a calça engomado* or "to iron the trousers" of your opponent.

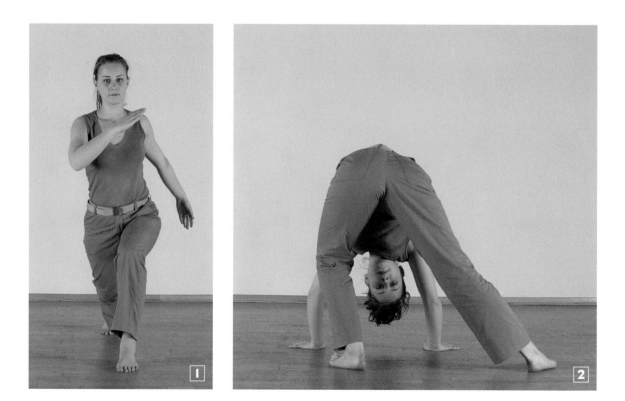

Pointers

Look through your arms and bend the support leg fully to make the kick as low as you can get it. It can rotate the full 360° degrees in a continuous circle as fast or as slow as your intention dictates. As with meia lua de compasso, the heel of the foot is the kicking surface.

Application in the jogo

The kick is extremely adaptable and can spin at your opponent from almost every conceivable angle, with lightning-fast changes of direction.

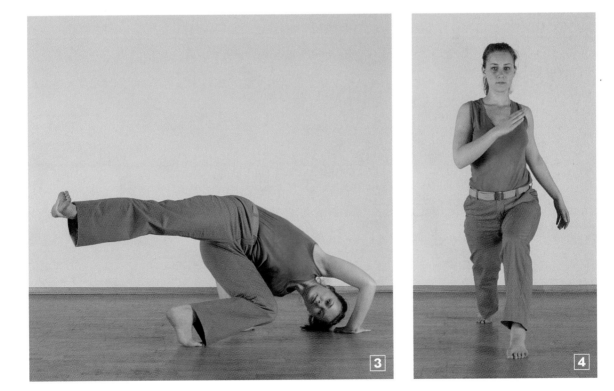

Intermediate Movements

34. Aú Cabeça no Chão

Movement

This is an aú with the head on the floor.

Pointers

There are many ways to begin this movement. In the photographs it begins with an esquiva lateral. The free arm extends out beyond her head and is placed on the floor, to give a secure base consisting of the palms of the two hands and the top of her head. In doing this yourself, as you go over, keep the legs down and to the front of your body so that you don't tip over backward. Having gone over in the aú, with one foot on the ground again, either stand up or do ground movements such as cocorinha, queda de quatro, queda de rins, or rolé to continue the game. It can also convert well into rabo de arraia.

Note: By keeping the weight distributed evenly between the head and two hands, there is never much pressure on the top of the head.

Application in the jogo

Aú cabeça no chão is good for moving around and changing direction on the ground. A player can drop into it from an aú normal, and from there also drop into an aú queda de rins or turn into a pião de cabeça. It is a useful following movement if the player has escaped under a rabo de arraia with a negativa lateral. Without raising the head from the ground the player may also continue with a moenda.

✦

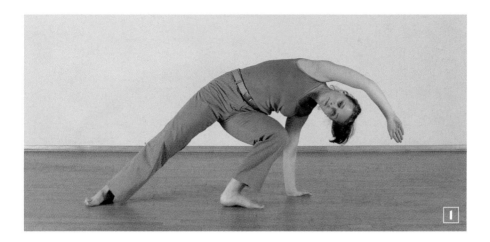

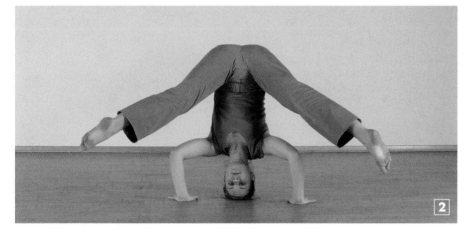

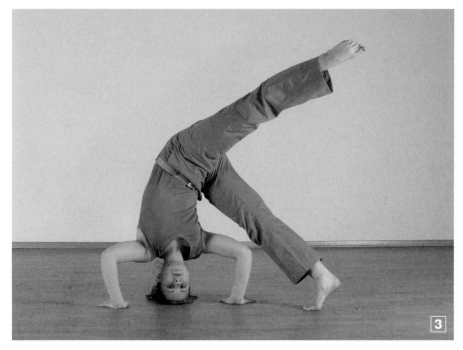

35. Aú Cruzado

Movement

This is similar to an aú normal, except instead of taking off from one foot and landing on the other, in aú cruzado you take off on one foot, cross it over to the front, and land on the same foot.

Pointers

As you cross the foot, keep your leg low to close your body to your opponent (fig. 3). In fig. 4 the player lands on the left foot, while still looking through his two arms, and then finishes off by twisting up into ginga, keeping the left foot where it is and the right leg to the back.

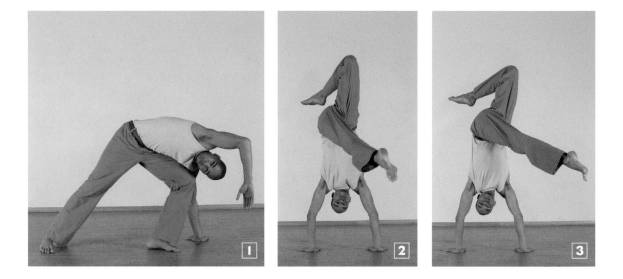

Application in the jogo

The extended leg in aú cruzado can either be straight, as in this set of photos, or bent and falling low in front of the player's body. The leg may pass over an opponent's movements while they are low on the ground, or stave off attacks during an aú, much like an aú compasso. In fig. 4, see how easily the right leg can swing around immediately for a rabo de arraia in the opposite direction to the aú cruzado without needing to switch feet. The right foot is also in a perfect position for a chapa de costas with only a slight shift in the angle of the player's body.

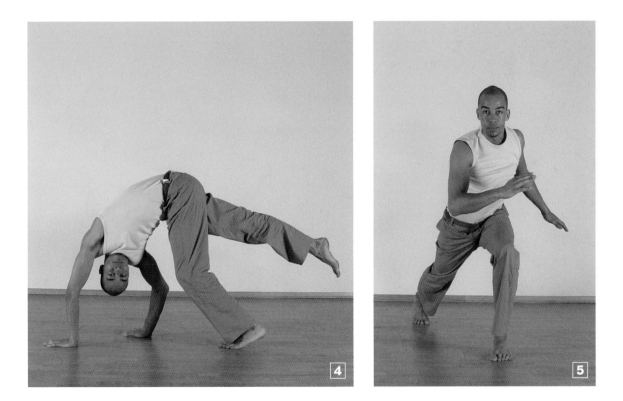

36. Corta Capim

(Capim Cortado)

Movement

Corta capim means "grass-cutter," because of the swinging rotation of the outstretched leg.

Pointers

Starting from an esquiva lateral (fig. 1), the player shifts his weight and the torso while swinging the outstretched leg in front of his body (fig. 2). As the leg swings around, the player leans forward, resting his weight on both hands (fig. 3), and finishes the movement by jumping his support foot over the rotating leg and continuing the swing around the back of his body (fig. 4). The full rotation is signaled when he reaches the fig. 1 position again. This can be repeated any

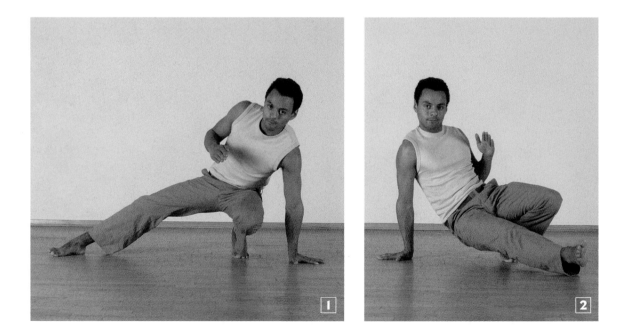

number of times so that the leg swings round and round in an uninterrupted circular motion.

To swing the leg round and round multiple times, it is not necessary to return to position 1 between swings, but rather to stay largely in the position depicted in figure 3 and just transfer weight from hand to hand and hop over the leg as it swings past. Get into a rhythm and let the momentum of the swinging leg help you through the movement.

Application in the jogo

If you stop this suddenly, with the front leg in negativa, it can be converted into all types of movements, for example, meia lua de compasso, rabo de arraia, or chapéu de couro. Corta capim can also be used as a foot sweep and converted into either a rasteira or alavanca. It can also be used to spin to the side of an opponent and position the player for an attack like vingativa.

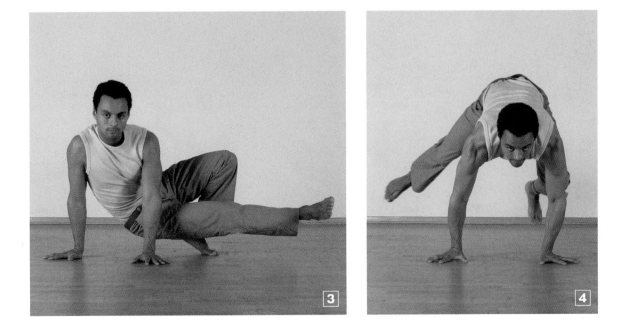

37. Aú Cabeça no Chão — Queda de Rins

Movement

In this queda de rins, the player turns over in an aú with the head on the floor and centers the hips to the front while dropping her waist onto her elbow.

Pointers

When you "fall on the kidney" in queda de rins, drop your waist down and press your elbow into the side of your waist. Do this simultaneously with landing one or two feet on the floor (as shown here in fig. 3), or it can be done before landing the feet (see movement No. 39).

Application in the jogo

This queda de rins technique can link one set of movements to another. Here the movement is an aú cabeça no chão directly hooking into the queda de rins, which in turn sets the player up to rise into ginga or continue into negativa, moenda, tesoura, relógio, or another aú cabeça no chão back in the other direction.

·❋·

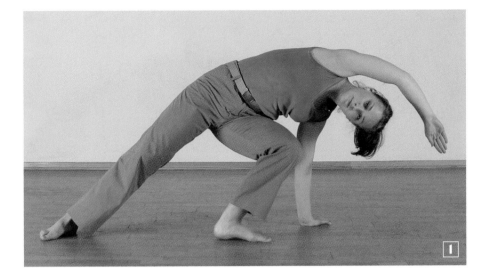

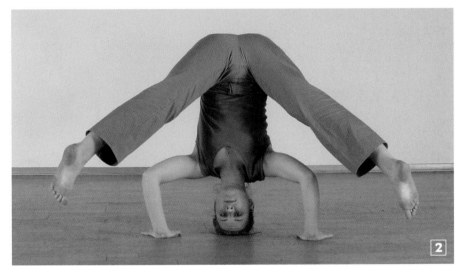

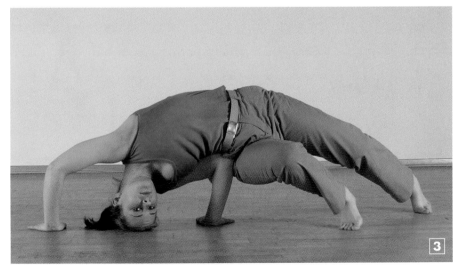

38. Esquiva Queda de Rins

Movement

This is an escape movement for a low game, tucking the elbow of the arm nearest the opponent into the waist (in the area of the kidney, hence the name "escape, falling on the kidney").

Pointers

As you lower yourself, keep your hips facing upward. Don't turn the hips to the side or this will change the type of esquiva you are doing. Position your hands as they are in the photo, thus providing the base, while you see your partner through the middle of your two hands. The knees are quite close together.

Application in the jogo

This is a movement you can fall into from an upright position, or from an already low position like cocorinha or resistençia. If someone did a low rabo de arraia, for example, you could face their oncoming kicking leg and drop beneath it in this esquiva. A good player can flip the two legs over his pivoting elbow and toward his own head to come out of this position.

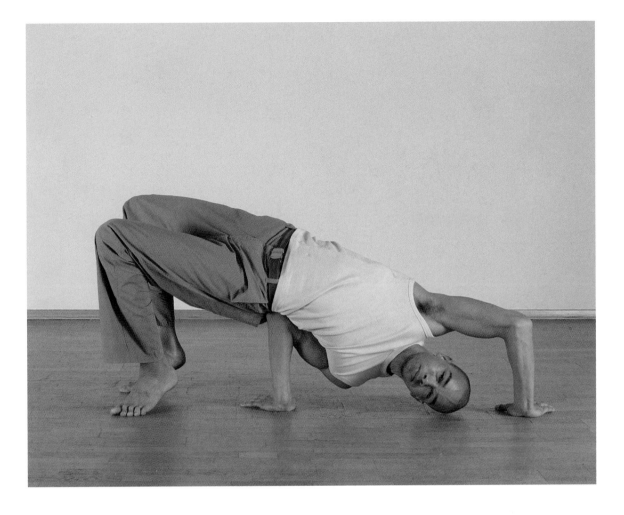

39. Queda de Rins

(MOVING)

Movement

The reason for calling this a "moving" queda de rins is to emphasize that the player has fallen into it directly from (for example) an aú normal **before** either of his feet have yet touched the ground.

Pointers

As you come out of your initial aú, whether it is normal or with head on the floor, control your body weight and drop lightly but directly down onto your elbow. If the movement is too fast or uncontrolled, hitting the queda de rins will be difficult, so practice by doing slow aú movements and dropping onto your elbow just as you turn over the halfway mark and begin your descent. As here, bend the legs and work on achieving a full queda de rins before your feet touch the ground.

Application in the jogo

This type of queda de rins has the same applications as the previous examples, with the additional advantage that it adds "flow" to the player's game and feels good to do. The player poised on his elbow here has the potential to roll out to the side, forward into negativa, around and back into moenda, or to tap one foot down to stop his momentum and push up into a bananeira.

⁕

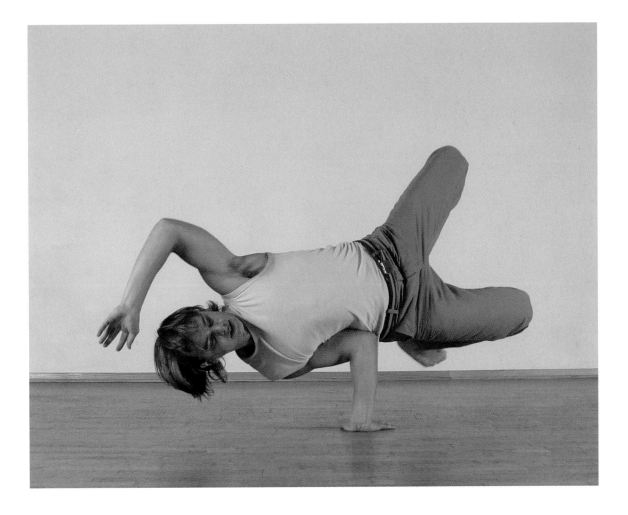

40. Bananeira Cabeça no Chão

Movement

Bananeira is generally a term referring to a handstand, though it can also mean a regular headstand. Here the player is doing a headstand, with her legs dropping down to the front.

Pointers

Use the hands to assist the balance, and practice tipping from one side to the other, bouncing on and off the toes of either foot to work on control.

Application in the jogo

Players often rest their weight on the head during the course of a game. This move could be converted into an escorpião or pião de cabeça, or the player could push up into a hand-balancing bananeira. She could also drop into queda de rins, turn for moenda, roll out into cocorinha or negativa normal, or shift around for a meia lua cabeça no chão.

⁕

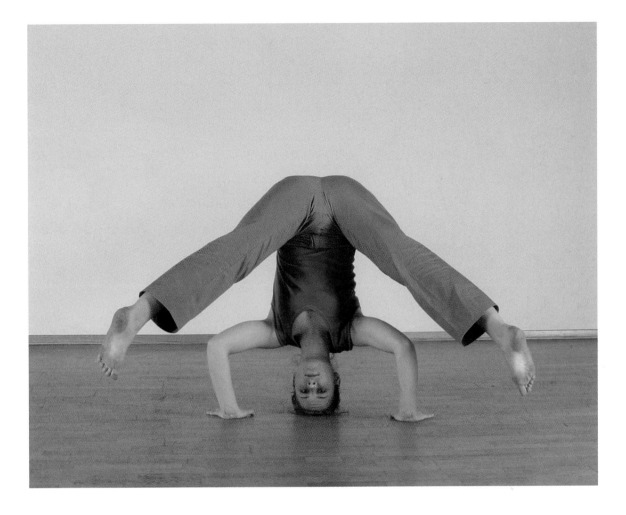

41. Bananeira

Movement

This movement is a handstand with the body open, in contrast to bananeira fechado (see below). There are many varieties of bananeira in capoeira, although rarely a handstand with the legs straight up in the air. Even here, in this open handstand, the legs are spread to create a symmetrical static pose, balanced on the hands.

Pointers

For stability here the player has locked out his arms and spread his fingers wide for a good base on the floor. In capoeira the player always looks forward through the arms, and never down at the floor. Hold your abs in firm, to create core balance throughout your body.

Application in the jogo

Some players do this bananeira and then twitch both legs rapidly to make their whole body vibrate. Other times, a player will do this handstand while their partner does a flying aú through their legs, although this is mainly for exhibitions in which the capoeira players are showing off their acrobatic skills. Alternatively, a player might present an open target like this to draw the other player into doing an attack technique, for which the player on the ground is already waiting and intends to answer with a counterattack such as aú batendo or aú quebrado.

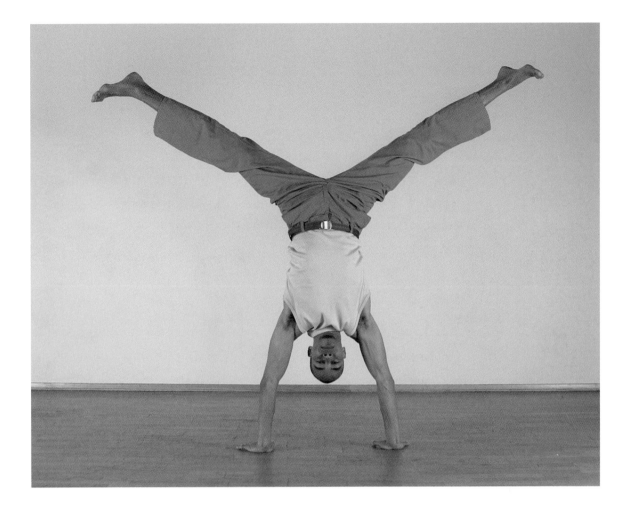

42. Bananeira Fechado 1

Movement

Bananeira is a handstand in capoeira, and fechado means "closed." This closed handstand uses the bent legs to protect the body of the player holding the bananeira.

Pointers

Writing about handstands, the capoeira player Greg Downey made an interesting comment in his book, *Learning Capoeira*. After experiencing difficulty with the balance, he was helped when his teacher said, "Just stand up." (Downey, *Learning Capoeira: Lessons in Cunning from an Afro-Brazilian Art,* Oxford and New York: Oxford University Press, 2005.) This is good advice. Imagining that your hands are feet, just stand up into the bananeira. Here, the arms are slightly bent at the elbow, though the fingers are well splayed for a strong wide base. The knees are very bent and the legs tucked in front of the body. Try to hold this position in training, and you can even do it balanced with your back against a wall for added support (although obviously there will be no walls available to lean against in the roda).

Application in the jogo

Going upside down is part and parcel of capoeira. It frees up both feet for kicks, and adds a whole different dimension to this unique fight-dance-game. A closed bananeira leaves the player less vulnerable. When you have developed a strong bananeira, it is possible to walk around on your hands, and even chase the other player while holding the inverted position and kicking.

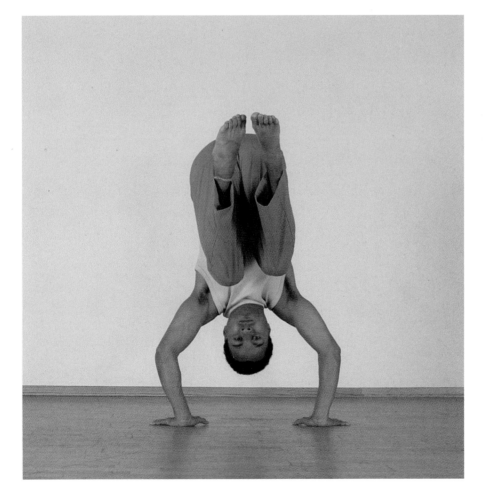

43. Bananeira Fechado 2

Movement

This is also a handstand, although in this case one leg is kept extended straight out to the front to ward off the advance of an opponent's attacks.

Pointers

Keep the front leg out straight and use the back leg to balance your body in the bananeira position. Always use one or another type of closed bananeira if you are playing someone you suspect will attack with head-butts. If you wait to discover their intentions by testing with an open bananeira, by the time you've found out it may be too late, as you will already be on your backside.

Application in the jogo

The same applications as for bananeira fechado 1 are relevant here. This movement may be easier for beginners to achieve, due to the effect of the back leg balancing out the movement.

✵

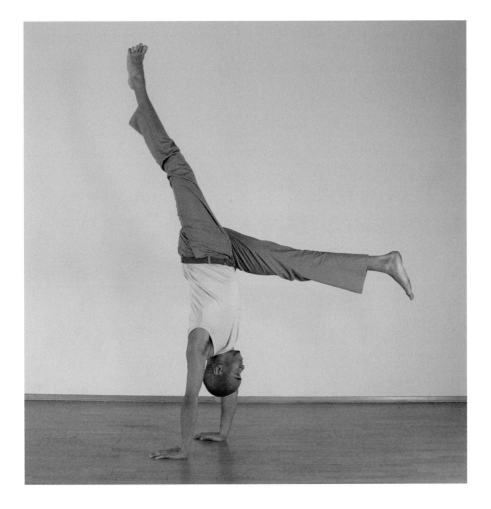

44. Moenda

Movement

The term *moenda* refers to the stone grinding wheel that was used for hundreds of years in Brazil to squeeze the juice out of sugar cane. This is a turning movement with the crown of the head on the floor. The player rotates her whole body from one side to the other without ever changing the angle of her head.

Pointers

This technique should be done smoothly in a continuous semicircle, preferably without stopping at any stage throughout its course. If you are stiff in your shoulders or back, practice this to loosen up those areas. Remember it is the body that turns around the head. When looking at your partner, don't turn away but rotate your body while looking in his or her direction the whole time.

Application in the jogo

In order to move with agility around the roda, it is vital that one's body can adapt to situations on the ground from every angle. Moenda is one of those movements that enables a player to weave imaginatively without being limited by stiffness in the spine. It is possible to begin a moenda and push up at the halfway point into a bridge (ponte), and then a walkover. A player can slip into moenda from other positions where the head is already on the floor. This isn't strictly a defensive or attacking move, but a means to what's referred to as *jogo bonito* or beautiful way of playing. It will help in both attack and defense, depending on the circumstances.

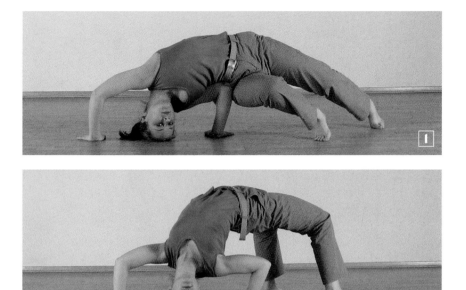

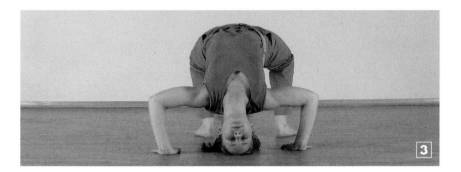

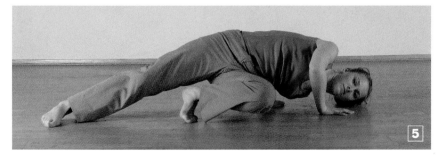

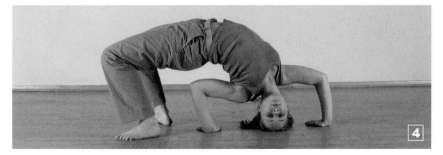

45. Aú Coisa

Movement

In fig. 1 the player reaches over and looks through her arms, as if preparing for aú normal. Doing the aú in fig. 2, the player holds a momentary bananeira with her knees pulled into her body, legs bent. She snaps out the aú coisa in fig. 3. After the kick, she pulls the knees back into her body and continues to complete the cartwheel (fig. 4).

Pointers

When kicking, keep the feet together, legs straight out and parallel to the floor, with the toes pulled back so the heel-end of the sole of the foot is the kicking surface. Pull the feet back quickly so that you don't fall forward but continue through to complete the aú.

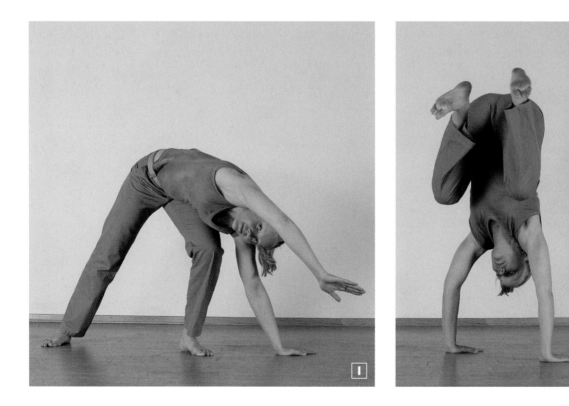

Application in the jogo

This is a surprise movement that looks exactly like a regular aú compasso until it is delivered. Because both feet kick from a solid foundation with the weight supported on two hands, it is also a powerful kick. Just holding the feet in a poised position (fig. 2) is a defense against a cabeçada. As with chapa de costas, the aú coisa doesn't need to make contact or even be fully extended toward your partner; it is there as a warning in case your opponent intends to deliver an attack against your aú.

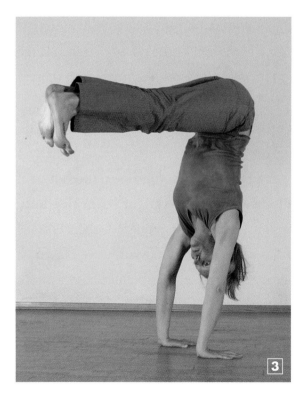

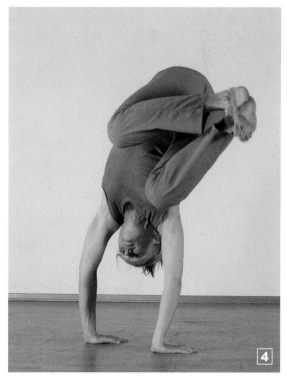

Aú Quebrado 2
(Bico de Papagaio)

Movement

Here is a variation on the bico de papagaio. The difference here is that the second leg is kept straight and doesn't tuck above the body.

Pointers

This technique is achieved in the same way as the previous kick, though note that here, the player's right arm locks in behind his kicking leg and he grasps his own ankle. The left leg, rather than tucking in, stretches out, including the foot, to balance the appearance of the technique. Recall that capoeira is also a game played to look good, so try to create symmetry with this move.

Application in the jogo

The application in the jogo is the same as for movement No. 46.

✦

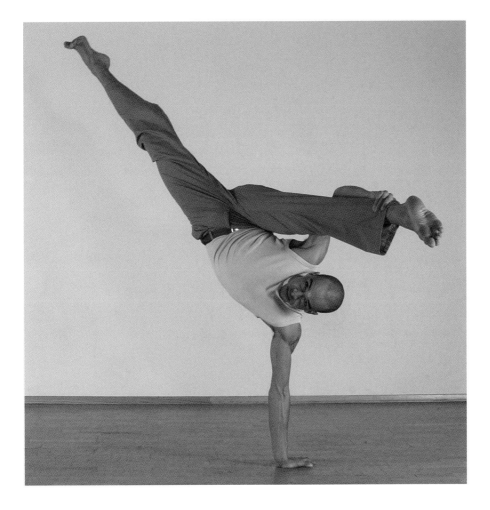

47. Aú Batendo

Movement

This is an aú with a powerful kick in a straight downward direction.

Pointers

The first foot to leave the floor leading into the aú will deliver the kick. Kick downward onto the target with the top of the foot. The second leg extends straight back to counterbalance the weight of the front kicking leg (see fig. 2). Having delivered the kick, continue the aú and land over on the other side (fig. 3).

Application in the jogo

This kick can be aimed downward onto a player doing cocorinha, resistençia, negativa normal, esquiva lateral, or negativa lateral, or to attack if a player advances for a cabeçada.

As a floreio, some players stop in the fig. 2 position, quickly switching the legs back and forth repeatedly. Some players even coordinate this with hopping up and down on their hands.

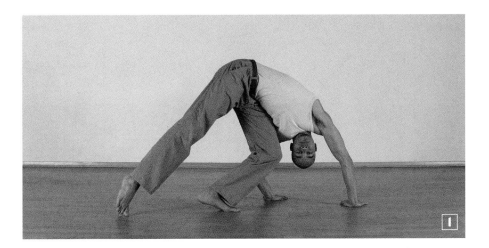

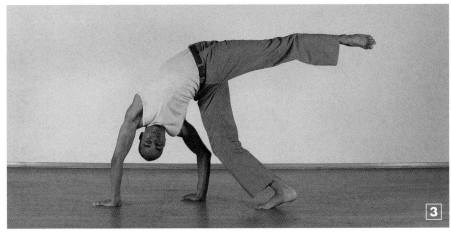

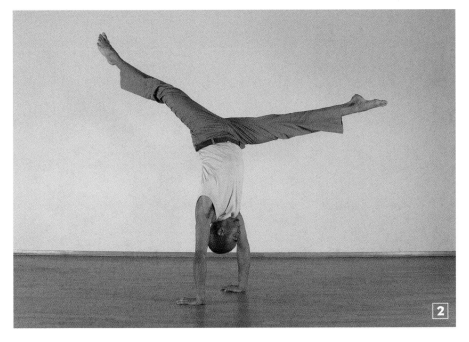

48. Chapéu de Couro

Movement

This movement is a kick that comes up from the floor, toward your partner with the leading leg. It's like a slice through the air, one leg after the other on the same trajectory.

Pointers

In fig. 1, the player begins in negativa normal to ready himself for the technique. In fig. 2 he hops strongly from his right foot, pushing up his hips, swinging the left leg up and forward across his body (with his left hand on the floor). To make this movement more efficient, start with your backside quite close to the support (left) hand, and feel that hand pushing into the ground, with the weight centered over it even as you do the kick. To gain the necessary momentum for a high and powerful kick, throw everything (the legs, torso, free hand, and head) over in the same direction for the kick.

Fig. 3 is the kicking part of the chapéu de couro. Fig. 4 is where this differs from the S-dobrado. The player doesn't reach back with his free hand to take it to the ground, but instead completes the kick with his free hand still off the ground. He lands on the kicking (left) foot. In fig. 5 the player brings his right foot back down to the ground, shifts the weight to his right arm, and is ready to continue play.

Application in the jogo

This kick can be used to surprise your partner by leaping at them directly from a grounded negativa position. It can be used to leap over a partner too. If you fall into negativa, it shows skill to bounce straight back up into a chapéu de couro without missing a beat.

❂

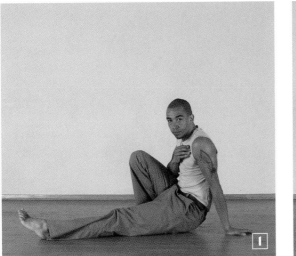

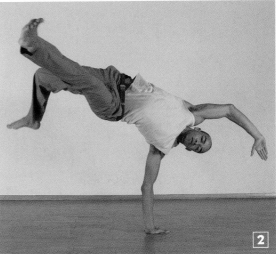

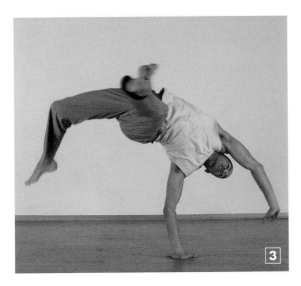

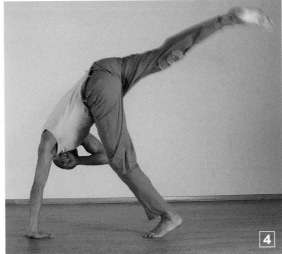

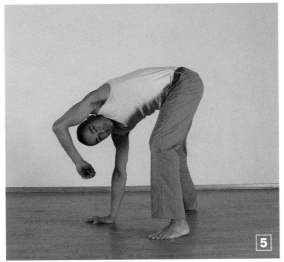

49. Meia Lua de Compasso—Queda de Rins

Movement

In this movement the player begins the meia lua de compasso in the same way as usual (fig. 1), but at the point of contact with the intended target, he drops into a queda de rins movement (fig. 2).

Pointers

Keep looking through your arms as you do the queda de rins, which means falling onto your elbow at the point where your kidney is situated (the side of your waist). Begin training this movement slowly to get the feel of it, and make sure the hand on the ground that is going to support your body weight is positioned with the fingers pointing away from you.

Application in the jogo

There is no single logical reason why you would particularly choose meia lua de compasso queda de rins above a rabo de arraia or other movement. It might be that you do it for aesthetic reasons, or that you feel you will continue out of the movement into a negativa normal and rolé, or spin around for a relógio. When you are playing a low game it is a good idea to try various queda de rins movements, including this one, to increase your choices within the jogo.

✦

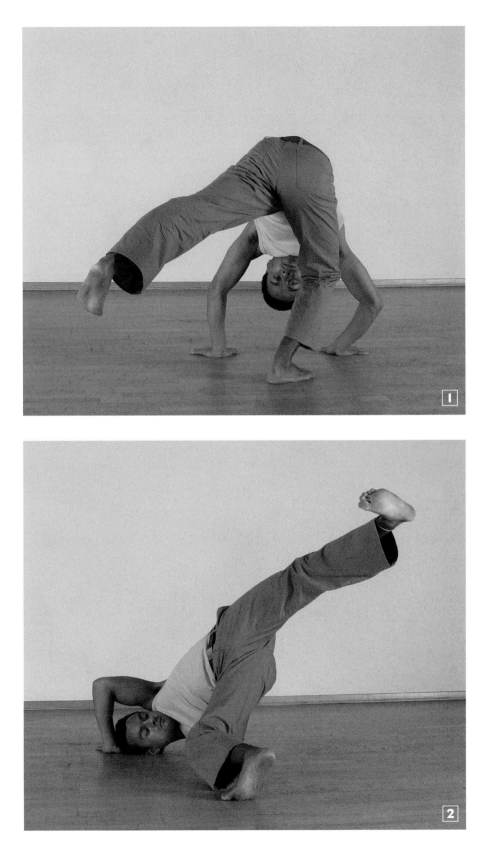

50. Meia Lua de Compasso sem Mão
(CHIBATA)

Movement

This kick is sometimes called *chibata,* because it is fast and explosive, like a whip. It is executed in a similar way to meia lua de compasso, except the hands are kept close to the body to protect the face of the person doing the kick.

Pointers

When doing this kick, the player lowers his head, swivels his hips, and forcefully spins his back right leg simultaneously (fig. 2), send-

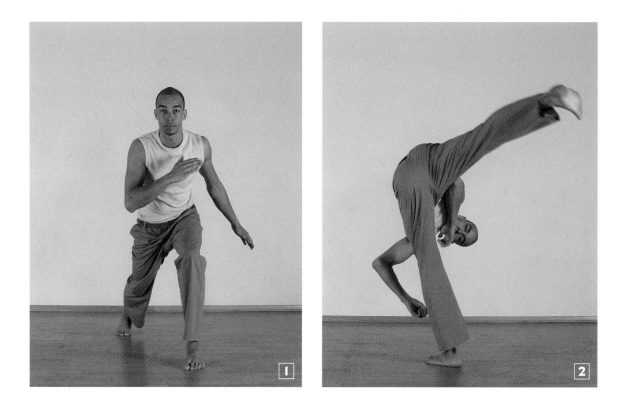

ing his heel toward his target. At the point where he reaches the target (fig. 3), his kicking leg is traveling at great speed, is very straight, his head is down and to the rear and, as you can see, protected by his arms. Make a point of not waving your arms about while doing this. After the kick is executed the player simply stands up again, returning the kicking foot to its original position.

Application in the jogo

This technique can be used in the same way as meia lua de compasso. It is such a fast and powerful kick that it should be used with caution, especially when playing with less experienced players, or when it is being done by less experienced players. The kick can inflict injury if it is done without due control and timing. Always be aware that your opponent might esquiva directly into your kick by accident.

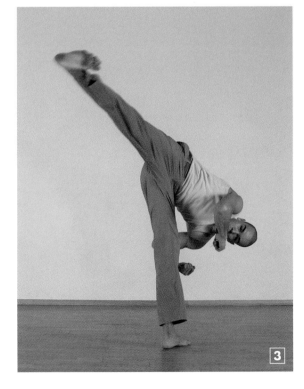

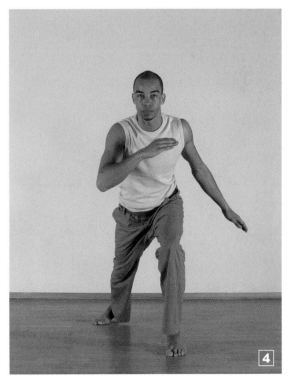

51. Meia Lua de Compasso Cabeça no Chão

Movement

This is a meia lua de compasso with the single difference that the head touches the floor on the way around.

Pointers

The head is on the floor to give possibilities to convert into many other cabeça no chão movements, though during this technique it only touches the floor briefly at the kick stage (180° from the start) of the movement. The weight is distributed evenly between the sup-

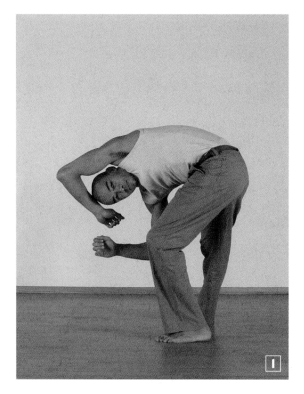

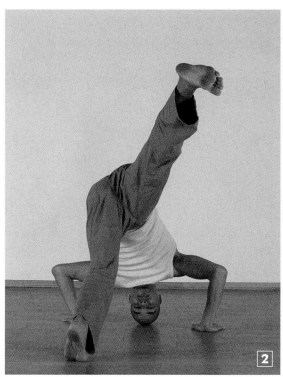

port foot and the two hands, and the head is not there for support during the movement.

Application in the jogo

This can be used as a meia lua de compasso kick, though due to the head being on the floor, the player has possibilities to stop at the kicking point and continue with other cabeça no chão movements or change direction.

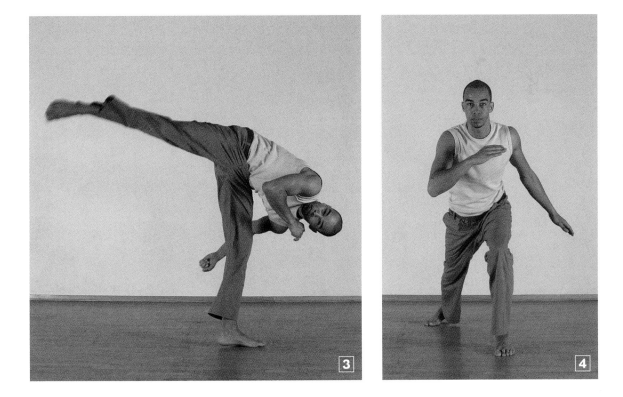

52. Alavanca

Movement

This technique is a turning, backward leg sweep, delivered low, either slowly and deliberately or powerfully and very quickly.

Pointers

This is an effective leg sweep. Timed right and hitting the outside heel or ankle of your opponent, it will usually put him on the ground. As you can see from the photos, the player turns without taking her eyes off the target. The drop-down transition that occurs between figs. 1 and 2 builds the momentum for the sweep. In fig. 3 the player's left leg (which was the rear leg in fig. 1) extends and circles around. This sweeping rotation continues right around to fig. 4. At this point the player could either just come up, so that she would then be in ginga position, or continue right around until the left leg is all the way at the back again. Note that the player keeps her hips down and tries to stay as low to the ground as she can for the alavanca.

Application in the jogo

This technique can successfully be used as a counterattack against all techniques which leave your opponent standing on one leg—for example, martelo, queixada, armada, chapa, etc. It can also be applied against a rabo de arraia in a low game. It is not always a good idea to hack your partner's leg out from beneath him as he plays, yet this movement is a very effective technique to mark the partner's kicks, bringing it just short at the point of would-be impact with his heels.

❁

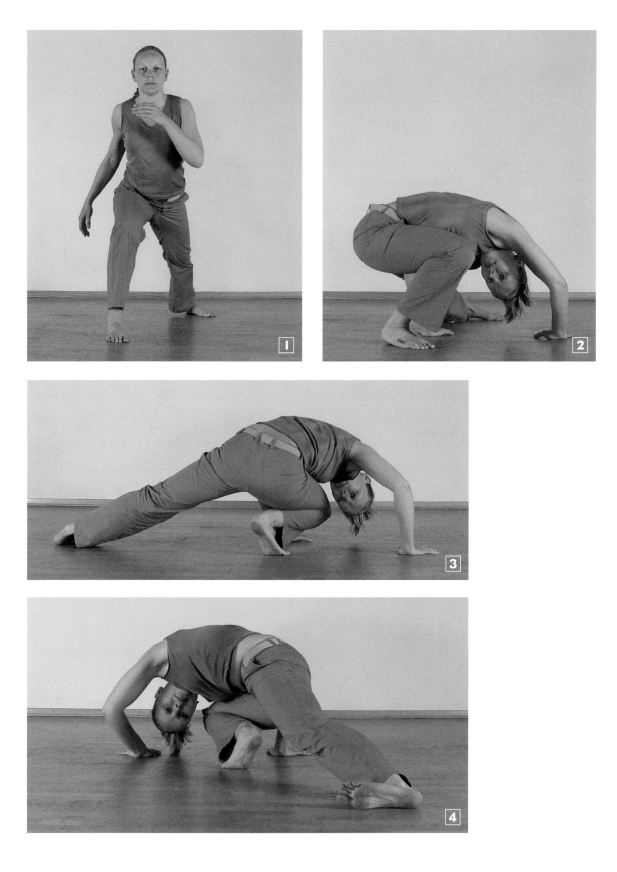

53. Encruzilhada

Movement

This leg sweep originated in the fighting game called *batuque*. The player turns quickly and drops into a squat, sweeping one leg around at speed to swipe the other player's leg (or legs) out from beneath them.

Pointers

Keep your eyes on your target area, which will be the back of the other player's ankle or ankles. Drop and spin simultaneously, relaxing the sweeping leg. Practice changing the arm that supports you on the floor (as happens between figs. 3 and 4 in the photos). There should be a smooth transferral of your weight from one hand to another on the turn. The encruzilhada shown in fig. 4 would enable the outstretched foot to hook around the back of the heel of another player. The technique is done so quickly that everything, ginga to the end of the sweep, happens in less than a single second.

Application in the jogo

This is classified as a *desequilibrante,* meaning it is designed to upset the balance of your opponent. You can fire this under kicks like armada, martelo, and even queixada if you are fast enough. At the end of the movement it is possible to continue around into a rolé, or double back into an aú. As with alavanca, this leg sweep is fully dependent on timing, and it works well as a "shown" movement to demonstrate what you could have done. As it requires a high degree of commitment to the turn for its effect, it's a sweep that should be practiced thoroughly until you're confident with it.

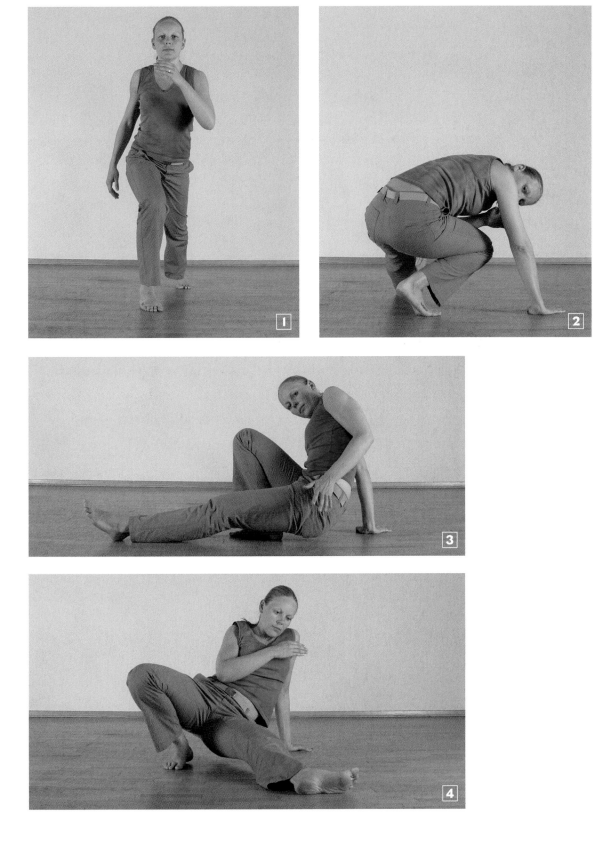

54. Rasteira 1

Movement

A rasteira is a "scythe," and while not the scythe of the Grim Reaper, it can reap serious effects on an adversary's body if it catches them mid-kick. This sweep cuts under high kicks in a swath. It's lightning-fast and very precise.

Pointers

A rasteira can be delivered with one, two, or no hands on the ground. The movement slices from fig. 1 to fig. 3 in a continuous, low, fast movement. The sweeping (right) foot would hook around behind the heel, or at the very highest, the ankle, of the other player. If the rasteira is delivered any higher it is no longer a foot sweep but a kick to the back of the other player's calf muscle. Timing is important with a rasteira, to ensure that it makes contact behind the adversary's foot. Often beginners, intent on dropping their partners, come

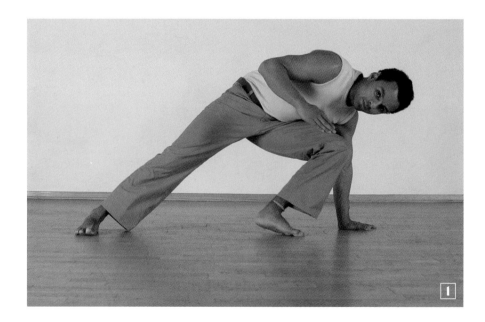

in too early and end up crashing shin against shin with the other player, bringing up a nasty bruise.

Note: Usually the rasteira makes contact with the heel and outside edge of the opponent's foot.

Application in the jogo

Rasteiras are fast, surprise movements that can upset the equilibrium of the other player. Often it is best to "show" the rasteira and not actually put the other player down, stopping it short at the exact moment it makes contact with the target area on the back of the opponent's foot. The rasteira is usually delivered to a player's support leg during the course of kicks such as armada, queixada, martelo de estalo, or any other technique that leaves them vulnerable on one leg. Rasteiras to the hands while a person is doing a bananeira or aú are treacherous movements that could result in serious injury to the other player, so they should be avoided.

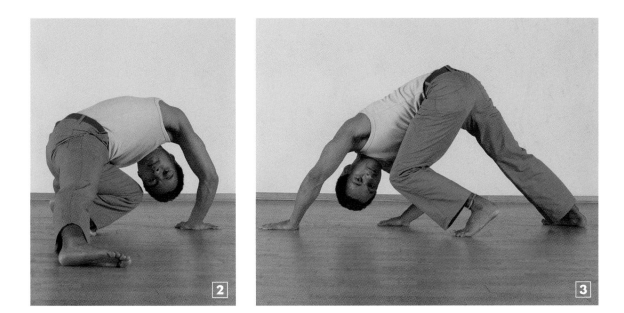

55. Rasteira 2

Movement

This rasteira snaps out rapidly from behind the player's own leading leg, making it especially surprising to the unsuspecting.

Pointers

Practice sliding smoothly and very quickly from fig. 1 to fig. 2. The sweeping (rear right) leg should dart out like a snake's tongue. Give it a snap as it extends to full length, which will propel your sweeping foot forward a short distance for extra "fetch" on your adversary's foot. After having delivered this rasteira, practice returning to your initial (fig. 1) position as quickly as you can, so that you are fast enough to go through the whole sequence before the other player even realizes what you have done.

Application in the jogo

This technique has similar application to the previous rasteira, although this is a more direct darting sweep from back to front, rather than a semi-circular motion. It is a technique that can be doubled up with an esquiva para trás and, as in the previous case, is useful against kicks such as martelo and armada, or even chapa and meia lua de compasso.

※

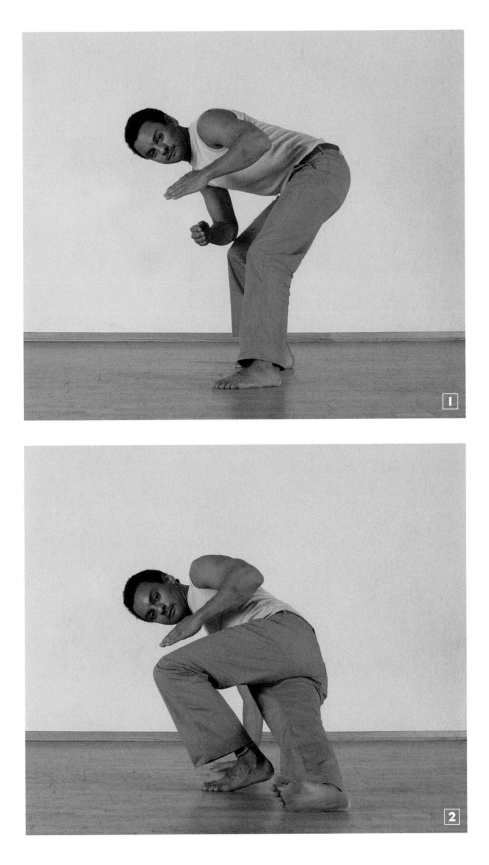

56. Joelhada

Movement

This capoeira technique was included in Mestre Bimba's published *Curso de Capoeira Regional* (*Course in Capoeira Regional,* an early instruction manual). It is a powerful front kick delivered with the knee.

Pointers

The knee comes straight up and forward like a battering ram.

Application in the jogo

In the Capoeira Regional course, the joelhada was featured as a defense against an *arpão de cabeça* (cabeçada) aimed at the solar plexus. It was simply driven up into the incoming face of the player delivering the head-butt. This is a technique that is well suited to self-defense, more so than in the capoeira game, in which violent, full-contact kicks are avoided. It is worth training some movements for self-defense from capoeira's large arsenal.

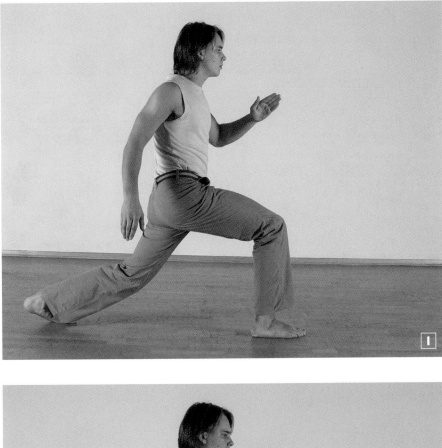

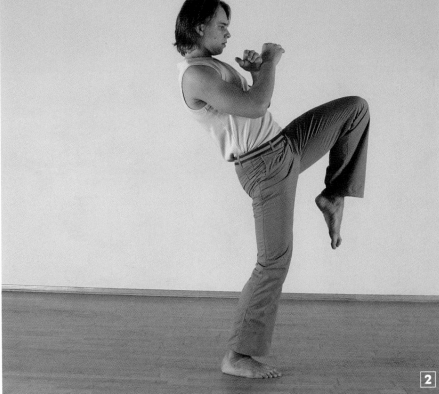

57. Galopante
(TELEFONE)

Movement

This is a fighting *golpe de mãos* (strike with the hands) that falls under the category of a traumatizing movement. The reason it is also called a *telefone* is clear, as it simply batters the ears with the heel of both cupped hands simultaneously.

Pointers

The arms are straight and the blow is delivered to the base of the ear with either one or (as shown here) two cupped hands.

Application in the jogo

Once again, this is a simple technique that has a very sound self-defense function, though it should only be used to "show" in a roda, as it is a dangerous blow with potentially serious physical effects that could even kill if delivered with force. The function of showing this technique, as well as the joelhada and hand strikes such as a *dedeira* (finger jab to the eyes) or *godeme* (a blow to the face with the knuckles of a back fist), is to warn another player about leaving his or her head too exposed to attack during ginga, as some players do.

⁕

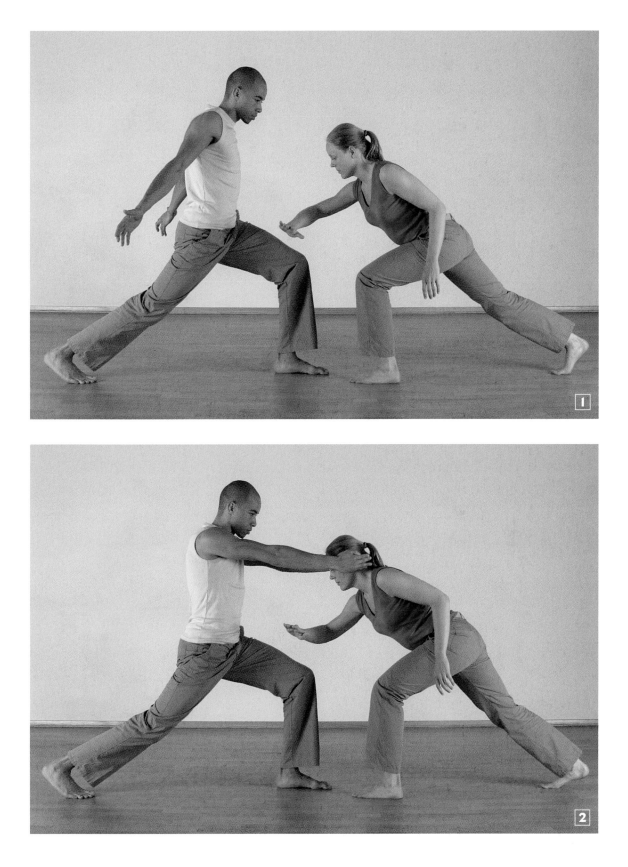

Advanced Movements

58. Aú

(ON THE FOREARMS)

Movement

This is an aú, though here the player uses his forearms on the floor instead of the hands.

Pointers

In fig. 1 the player drops low into a semi esquiva, with his hands already in position above his head, fists loosely clenched **before** he goes over for the aú (fig. 2). As you turn over keep the chin well tucked in, so that it is the forearms that take the weight of your body (to differentiate this from aú cabeça no chão). Get enough momentum on the turn to take you back up to your feet again. If you have difficulty finishing the movement off, slightly straighten your arms at the point when your feet hit the ground, to push up back onto your feet again.

Application in the jogo

Playing on the forearms is a great style of playing jogo no chão. As well as being fun to do, it will occasionally work in your favor to out-fox your opponent, who may not have seen it done before.

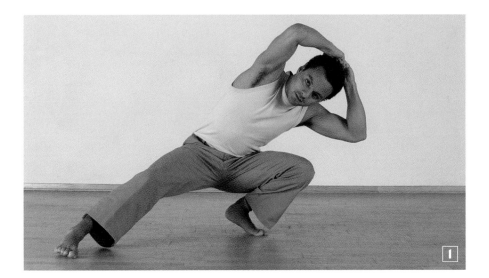

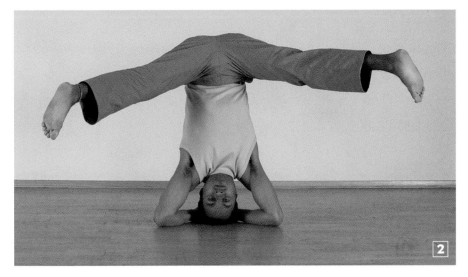

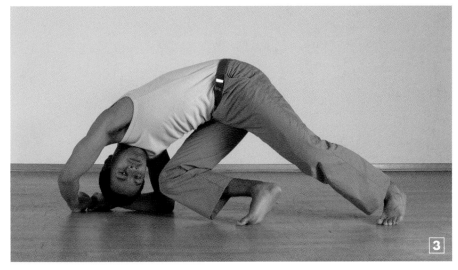

59. Aú Chibata

Movement

This movement is sometimes called *compasso*. It is a kick with the heel, built on the momentum of the body twisting and spinning one leg heel-over-head, so it whips down onto the intended target with great force and speed.

Pointers

In this set of photos the player will deliver the chibata with his right foot. In fig. 1 he begins with his right kicking foot at the back and is preparing his arms and torso to twist to the right. In aú chibata you will always twist and leap to the right if you intend to kick with the right foot, and to the left if you intend to kick with the left foot.

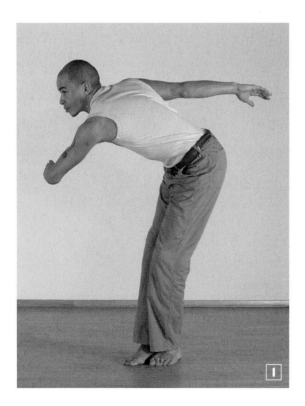

As he twists, he also jumps upward, bringing his straight right leg over his body and bending his left leg. He takes the weight of his body on his left support arm as the right leg whips over the top of the spin (fig. 2). Keeping his left hand down for support, he completes the move by falling onto his left foot. The right foot slams down on the target. Note that the right heel does not hit the floor, as it might damage the floor (or the heel).

Make sure you do this as a leap and not as an aú normal falling into a negativa normal.

Application in the jogo

If this heel kick makes contact with a target at full force, the victim will remember the result for a long time, so go easy and learn to control the kick before using it in the roda. The aú chibata is useful for leaping over your partner, and it is even more impressive if you can leap high off two feet and postpone the moment when you whip down the kicking leg for as long as possible. The aú chibata is often used as a leap and a shown movement, pulled before it hits the opponent. Because of its violent force, rarely is it appropriate to actually kick someone with this technique in the roda. To come out of the movement the player could transfer the weight to his right hand and continue on his way with a rolé to the right.

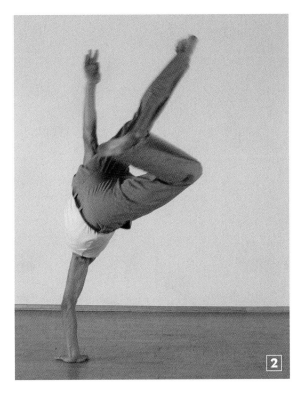
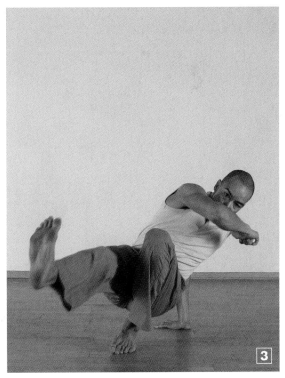

60. Aú sem Mão

(AÚ MORTAL)

Movement

Literally, this is an "aú no hands" or a cartwheel done in mid-air (aerial cartwheel).

Pointers

As in figs. 1 and 2, swing your hands and torso down and up in a U movement, using your waist as your pivot point. This is the "dip" phase of the movement. At the end of the U-movement (fig. 3), throw yourself up, kicking your back leg up for the aú rotation. The front leg pushes up to give you height. As you go over (fig. 4) pull your arms in to get more rotation, and attempt to keep legs splayed and straight as you can. Land as in fig. 5, on the front leg. (Because you've spun over in mid-air, the front leg has changed, so that in the photos the player has launched off the left foot and landed on the right foot.)

Application in the jogo

This is an exciting and spectacular flying movement which is fun to do in a fast and acrobatic game. Because you are facing the front and can do this without a run up, it is possible to do this acrobatic movement while remaining fully engaged in the game. In modern capoeira, old-timers sometimes criticize the use of acrobatics for acrobatics' sake, saying that the showy moves have no connection to the jogo de dentro. Aú sem mão can be played within jogo de dentro and is a useful movement to add to your arsenal. You can also enter the roda with this technique, though this would probably be done when the roda has warmed up and not in the early games.

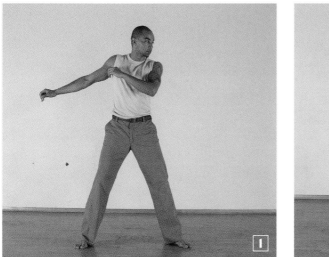

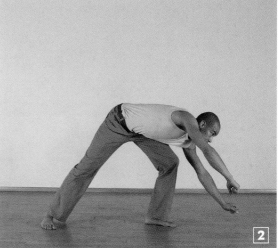

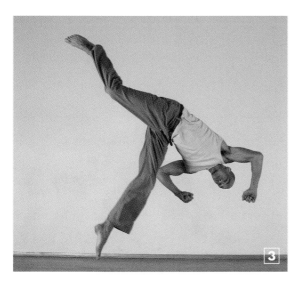

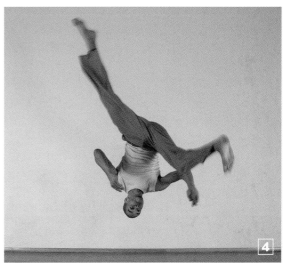

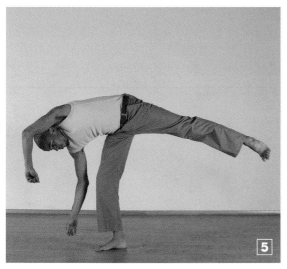

61. Aú Quebrado

(ON THE FOREARM)

Movement

Aú quebrado, whether done on the forearm or on one hand, involves the kicking foot smashing forward and inward, while the other foot tucks in with a bent knee. It is a kick always delivered upside down.

Pointers

A regular error is to attempt to kick the leg out to the side. In the photo it appears that the player is kicking to the side, but the reality is a forward kick. Kick into position as soon as you put the weight onto your forearm, or you will lose balance. Kick forward and inward with a straight leg until you reach the point where your leg is fully extended, then bounce or "unkick" back through the same angles, as if you were playing a video recording of the movement in reverse. The motion of the kick and the whip back into the original position take you back onto your feet. The movement is done smoothly and quickly.

Application within the jogo

Aú quebrado is a kick that can be used as an attacking movement or a floreio. Many techniques in capoeira that are normally done on the hands can also be done on the forearms—for example, aú normal, aú compasso, rolé, etc.

✦

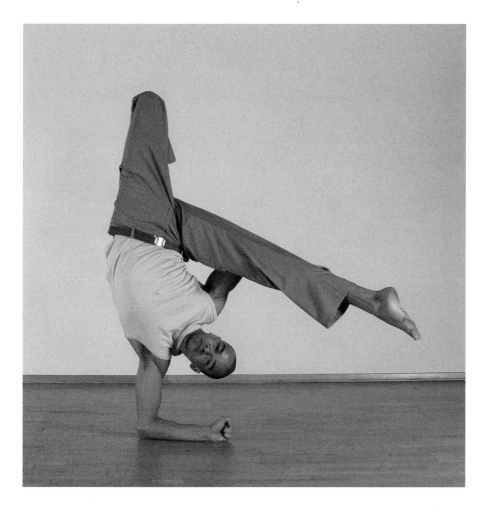

62. Aú Quebrado 3

Movement

This is an aú quebrado with a diffference in that the player, having placed the left hand on the floor, kicks up both legs together.

Pointers

Once secure on the support hand, twist the body, straighten the legs, and kick both legs together, as if attempting to hit your own chest with your knees. With the free hand, reach up and touch the toes at the top of the movement. As soon as you have touched your toes, snap the legs back into their original position.

Application in the jogo

This is an undisguised acrobatic floreio, which makes for an interesting inclusion in the jogo. After the technique has been realized, the player can bring the legs back down into an esquiva lateral, or could bring one (the left) down straight, and the right bent to land in negativa.

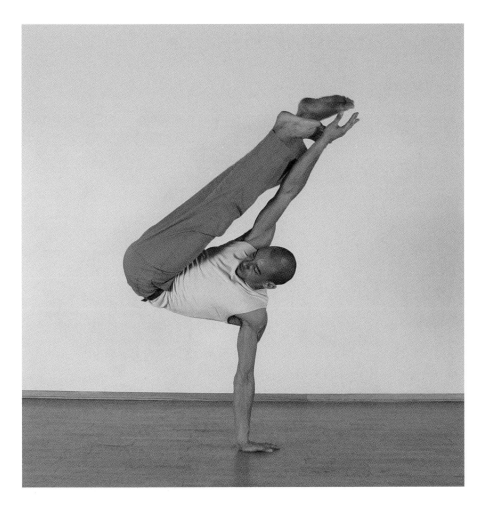

Aú Quebrado 4

Movement

This technique also kicks down with the two feet, though here they go much lower, in a basic approximation of a regular bico de papagaio, only doubled, so that both legs are moving in toward the player's own chest. His free arm is held straight up between the two knees, though it could just as well wrap around the legs, or go up behind or in front of them.

Pointers

Practice the regular aú quebrado 1 until you feel confident with taking your weight on one hand and controlling the technique, as well as the exit from it. In this technique, once the legs have reached their full extension, snap them forcefully back out of the movement to flip back to your original position. Keep your body weight centered directly over the support hand. If you tilt over too far, you'll tip forward, bringing the leg down to the ground in front of your chest, which is feasible though not as skillful.

Application in the jogo

This could be used as a two-footed kick by a skilled player, although it is more likely to fit the category of floreio and be applied as such.

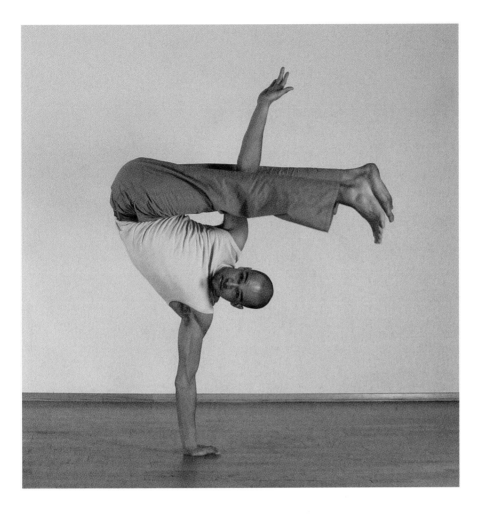

63. Pião de Cabeça

Movement

This is a head spin.

Pointers

Try to enter and exit the spin facing your partner. In the heat of the moment it isn't always possible to come out of the spin directed at your partner, though orient yourself and re-enter the game as quickly as possible. If you collapse, try to land on your hands and feet (in a push-up position) rather than flat on your back. In figs. 2, 3, and 4 the player brings up his legs and chops them in a scissors movement to begin the spin. In figs. 3 and 4, the player brings his right leg from the back, switching it to the front to begin spinning to the right.

During the spin itself, the player brings his legs together and straight upright (fig. 5). As the spin slows or he begins to lose balance (whichever comes first will vary from person to person or technique to technique), the player brings his hands down to the ground and his legs part in a scissor again (fig. 6). Then he brings his legs down to the floor to face his partner (fig. 7). You can train by doing quarter turns with the hands and legs kept to the front of your body.

Application in the jogo

Unlike the head spin sometimes done by b-boys in break-dancing, a capoeira head spin isn't meant to go on for very long. It has to fit with the action of the game, so capoeiristas don't train to spin around for dozens of rotations. Players usually pião de cabeça for as long as the initial momentum of the spin rotates the body (usually between one and four times). Rarely will players use their hands to continue spinning longer.

This falls into the category of a floreio to demonstrate a player's skill and daring. Excepting competitions, in capoeira players don't "win" by scoring points, but they can score personal victories in the eyes of their peers by playing with imagination, skill, or clever strategy. Even humor can add to the quality of some players' games. Moves like pião de cabeça are brilliant to do for the sheer fun of doing them.

❋

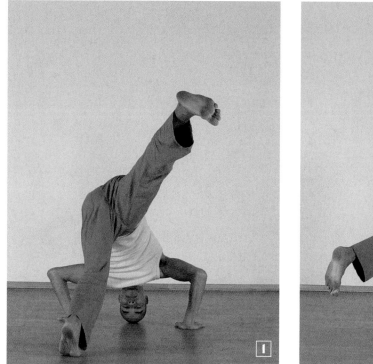

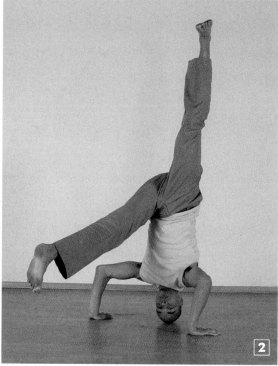

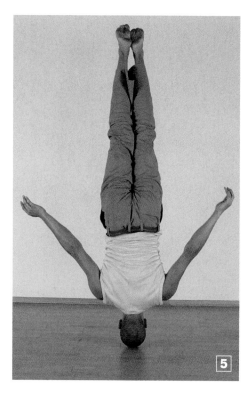

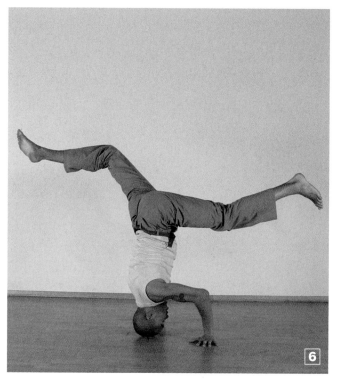

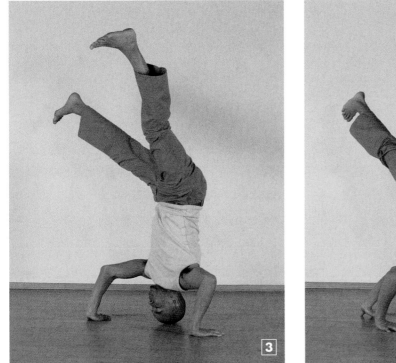

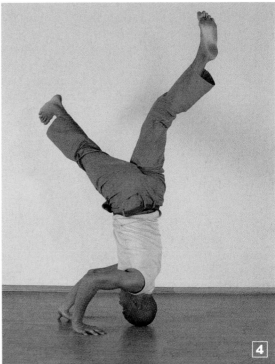

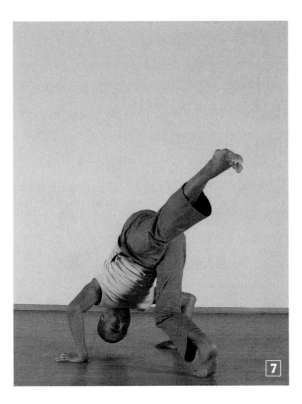

64. Pião de Mão

Movement

Pião de mão means to "spin on the hand." There is no one way to do the pião de mão, as some players go up into a handstand and then rotate by crossing their hands continually. Another way is to kick around rapidly as if doing a meia lua de compasso, then to lift the support leg and switch hands, which will begin the spin. In the movement here, the player switches hands just once (between figs. 1 and 2), after having built up enough momentum with his initial kick-off (fig. 1), then raises both legs vertically and spins on the heel of his support hand (fig. 3).

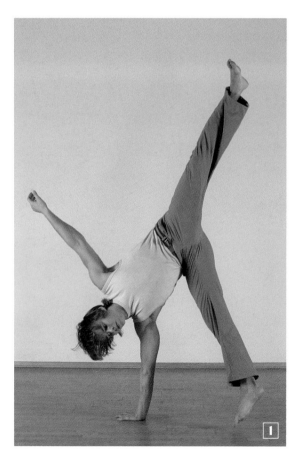

Pointers

In fig. 1, the player kicks off for the spin with a big movement (in this case a turning aú, although it could also have been a meia lua de compasso). He is beginning on his right hand. In fig. 2 he switches the weight onto his left hand and continues the spin. In fig. 3, he straightens out his legs, centers his weight directly over his support arm, and spins for as long as possible (which will vary from player to player). Try initially to work on the kick-off and weight shift from one hand to another so that you are attempting an aú with a single 360° turn. This in itself is a nice-looking movement. After you've got this, build up speed and try for more rotations. Keep the weight centered over the heel of your hand-wrist and up your straight arm; otherwise you will come down prematurely.

Application within the jogo

The pião de mão fits right in with games of capoeira characterized by turning kicks and rotational movements. It is also possible to drop out of it into negativa, resistençia, or other ground movements with speed. The only drawback to this type of movement is that in the middle of it the player is left vulnerable to attack, particularly to cabeçada, so be aware of this as you do it, and if you are with a tricky opponent, even more so.

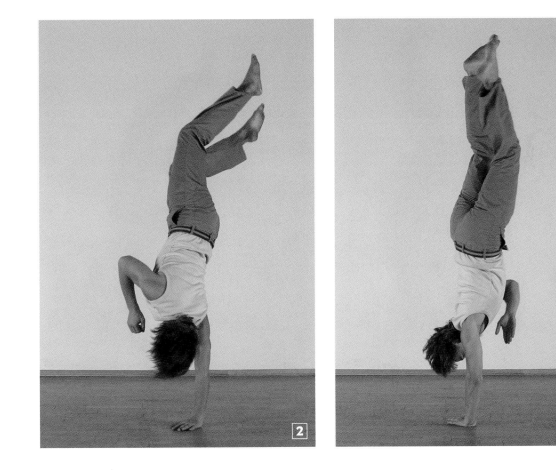

65. Escorpião

Movement

This is similar to a bananeira, though here the back is arched, the chin in, head forward, the chest thrust out, and the legs arching back to create a balanced position imitating a scorpion's stinging tail.

Pointers

Once you feel stable in the regular bananeira, push your chest forward and let your legs slowly arch back behind you. Keep them extended and don't bend them to make them reach down lower. The angle you can form with your legs in relation to the floor is largely determined by the flexibility of your shoulders and lower spine, so don't try to push things.

Application in the jogo

Static balances in the game of capoeira are done to demonstrate strength, flexibility, and body control. They can be set as a trap, to draw an opponent toward you (for a downward kick like aú batendo, for example), or simply to challenge them to show their own balance, or to answer a balance.

If you are playing a close game, particularly with an opponent you don't trust very much, escorpião is probably a move to avoid.

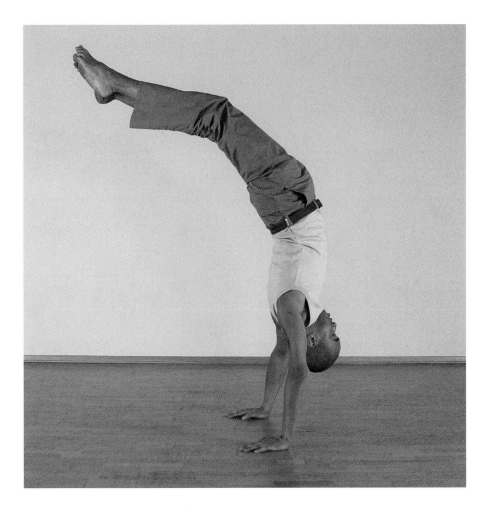

66. Escorpião Cabeça no Chão

Movement

In this movement the player is inverted and balanced on a triangular base of head and two hands outstretched behind him. From that base, he lowers his legs toward the ground, bending at the base of his spine to make the shape of a scorpion.

Pointers

From a regular headstand shoot both hands back simultaneously, so that the arms are fully extended. Let the legs fall back slightly to create the balance. From here, slowly begin to lower the legs. Don't bend the legs in an attempt to take the feet closer to the ground; the legs should be as straight as you can get them. Thrust your chest out as you hold the position, and make sure you are balanced on the top of your head.

Application in the jogo

This type of escorpião has the same applicability as the previous technique.

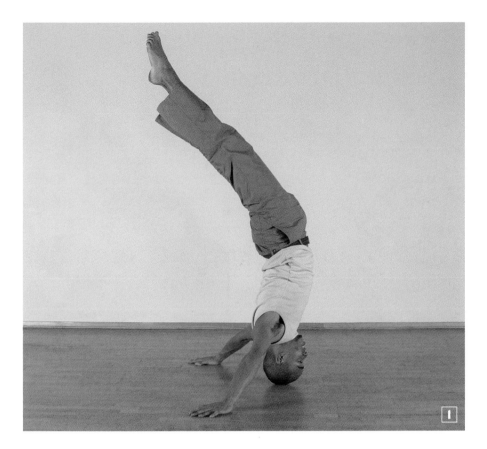

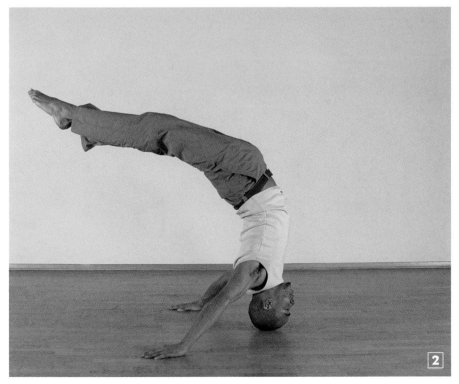

67. Invergado

Movement

This is a bananeira with both legs extended out in front and parallel to the floor.

Pointers

Keep the elbows locked out and the legs very straight. Tilt the head forward, looking at your two feet. Thrust the chest toward your thighs, and bring the thighs toward the chest. Try to hold this position.

Application in the jogo

As well as being a defensive bananeira, this is also a demonstration of body control and balance. There is a place for these kinds of demonstrations within capoeira, both in shows for the non-capoeira-playing public and as a good-humored competitive challenge to the opponent, to see who has the best physical dexterity.

※

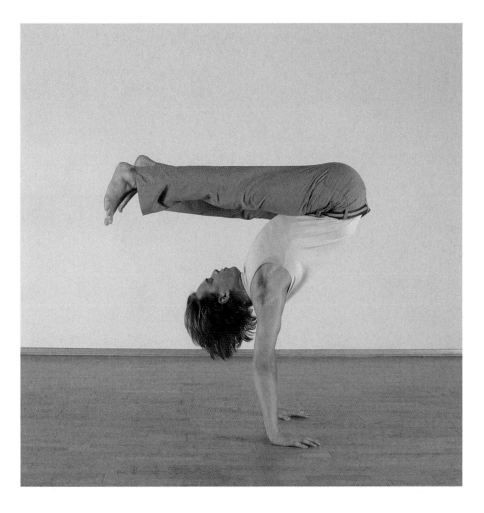

68. Aú Espinha

Movement

This is an aú "spine." During the movement the spine is rotated so that both hips are facing forward in the direction of the movement, rather than laterally to the movement (as in aú normal).

Pointers

Note that the player executing this movement launches off from his front right foot (fig. 2) and finishes up landing on his right foot again (fig. 5). The swing of his (right) leg over his body through the phases 3, 4, and 5 creates the momentum for the aú. In fig. 4 his weight is over his hands and he keeps his torso and hips centered over the movement. In fig. 5, the player drives his hips forward into the recovery (fig. 6). He does not collapse them upon landing (which would put him in a resistência). Beginners sometimes like to try espinha landing on two feet rather than one. This is an acceptable compromise but only remains aú espinha if you land with the hips forward and do not collapse them into resistência position.

Application in the jogo

Aú espinha gives mobility around the roda. Many players do it as much as aú normal. It can be done forward or backward. To do it backward you would literally reverse the process of the movements, as if you were working from fig. 6 back to fig. 1. The espinha can propel you forward, or you can aú espinha in the same spot repeatedly, without moving forward. This movement increases possibilities to move freely in the game, from whatever angle your hips or torso happen to be at a given moment.

✺

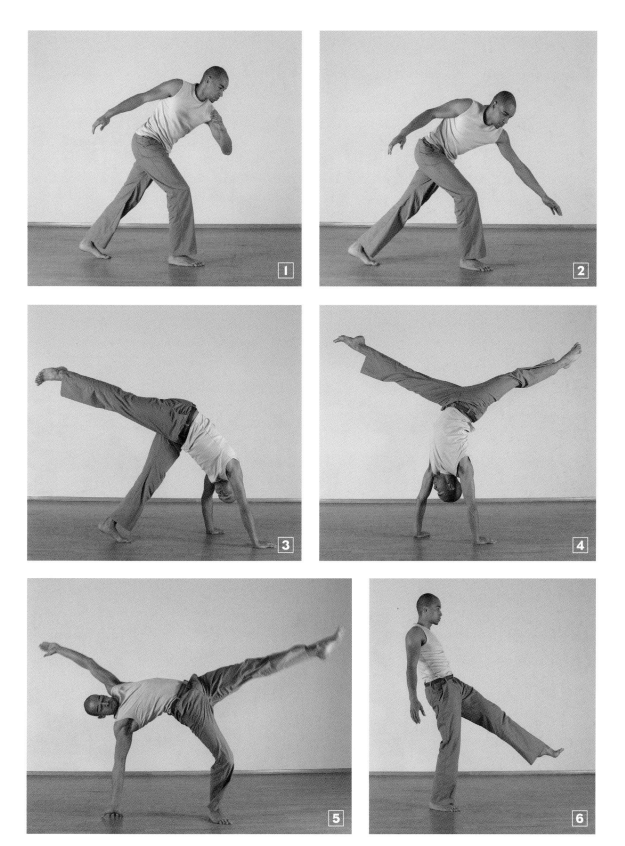

69. Rabo de Arraia

(FROM A HANDSTAND)

Movement

Don't confuse this kick with a low meia lua de compasso. It is common in capoeira for movement names to have regional variations. The movement involves kicking up into a handstand, but instead of looking forward through the middle of your arms (as in bananeira), the player extends his neck and whips one leg out for the kick over his back.

Pointers

In the picture, the player is kicking with his right leg and tucks the left in. This is optional, as the leg that is not kicking can be stretched out to help with balance. The height of the kick depends on where you are aiming. In fig. 1, the kick is aimed high, at an upright player's head height. In fig. 2, the player kicks directly ahead, parallel to the floor, with the sole or heel end of the sole of his foot.

Application in the jogo

The usefulness of this kick lies in the unexpected angle from which it is delivered. If you are crouched on all fours and looking forward at your partner (like a cat), they are not expecting a kick coming straight at them over the top of your head.

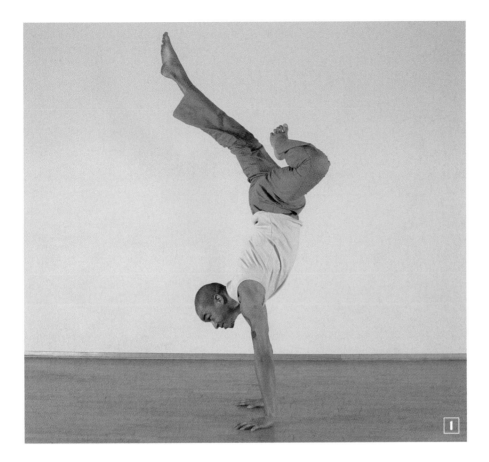

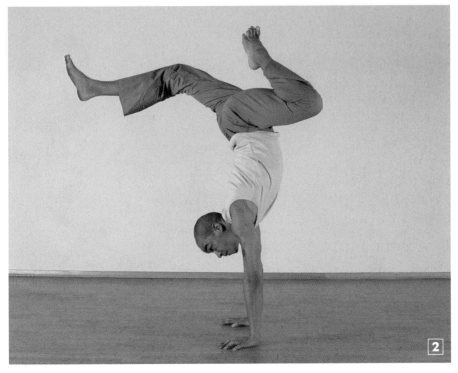

70. Macaco

Movement

Macaco is a flip backward, one hand at a time, with both feet and legs held quite close together, jumping off and landing on two feet.

Pointers

The starting position for macaco is resistência (fig. 1). The player squats on their haunches with one hand placed on the ground at their side. The player bounces off from both feet, throwing the hips and reaching one hand back over his head (see fig. 2).

The higher you can drive your hips at the start of the movement, the easier it will be to flip over. When doing macaco, always begin with the hand on the floor in your opponent's direction so you can still see them as you do the movement.

Make sure your other (outstretched) arm also goes over slightly in that direction; otherwise you may land flat on your back. The head arches back in the same direction as the outstretched arm (fig. 3). Both hands go to the ground (fig. 3). Both legs flip over together (fig. 4) and land still together (fig. 5).

Application in the jogo

Macaco is a versatile and elegant movement which can be an extension of many esquivas. In this example, it is an extension of the esquiva "resistência," though it can be delivered equally well straight after a negativa normal, a cocorinha, or an esquiva lateral. Use macaco for quick evasive changes of direction, done with panache and athleticism.

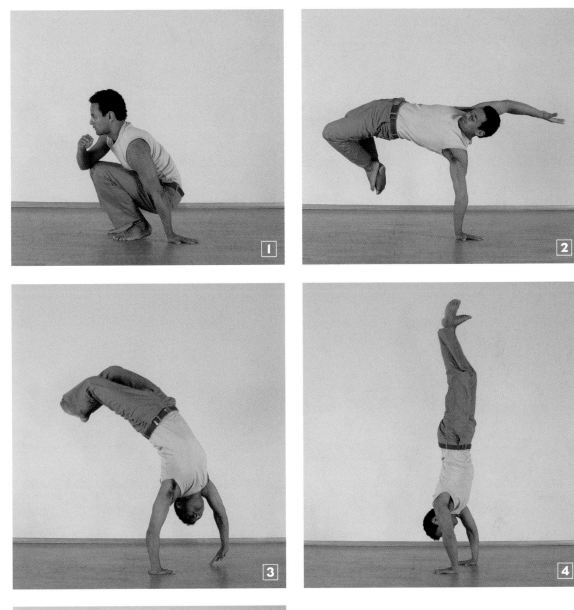

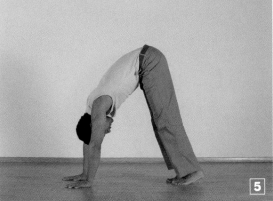

71. S-Dobrado

(S-Macaco)

Movement

This movement is similar to a regular macaco, but it is launched by a swing of one leg in a kind of S-shaped loop. In figs. 1, 2, 3, and 4 we can see a directional change. In fig. 1, the player is leaning over the left leg, as if he's about to launch off for an aú to his left. In figs. 2, 3, and 4, however, he swings the right leg around and throws it upward in S-dobrado in the opposite direction. In figs. 5 and 6, the player follows through with his left leg, making a switch at the top of the movement, so he lands once again on his left foot.

Pointers

Lead with the hips as you go over in the S-dobrado. Between figs. 3 and 4, the player has pushed off forcefully from his support (left) foot, swung the right foot, and thrown up the hips to gain height. Note that S-dobrado is similar to chapéu de couro but is differentiated from that technique by the swinging leg going straight over the player's body at the top of the movement, and the fact that both his hands touch the ground (fig. 5).

Application in the jogo

This is a great technique for fast changes of direction, and it is aesthetically a winner. It converts directly from esquiva lateral or, as shown, can be done to fool the other player about your intended direction within the game. The S-dobrado can also be used as an attack technique (see No. 72, next).

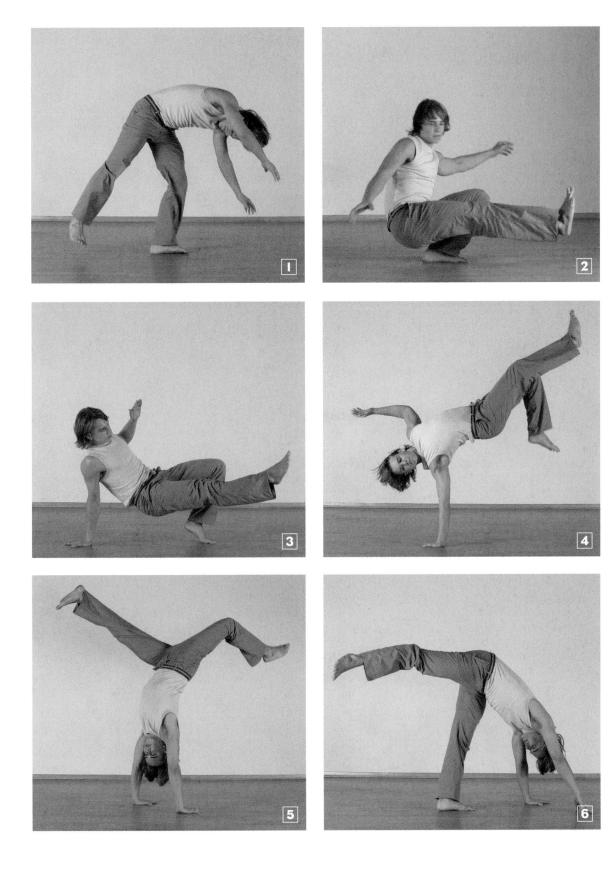

72. S-Dobrado 2

Movement

This movement begins and ends in the same way as No. 71, though here, in fig. 2, the player swings out with a kick forward, even as his body is flipping over in the S-dobrado/macaco technique.

Pointers

Practice kicking to the fore of your body while continuing to arch back and reach over to place both hands on the floor. Land on the same foot that you push off in the first place (here, the left foot).

Application in the jogo

This is a useful defense if someone decides to move forward toward you with cabeçada or another attack during the course of the S-dobrado.

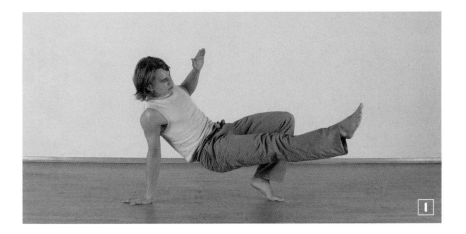

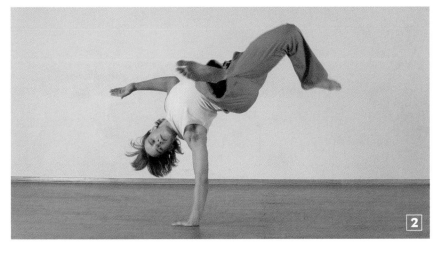

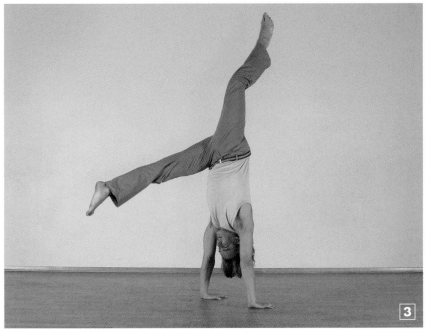

73. Mola

Movement

Mola means "spring" in English. This is one of the few movements in capoeira that involves touching anything other than the hands, feet, or head on the floor. Mola is a spring from the back of the shoulders to the feet.

Pointers

Beginning in cocorinha position (fig. 1), the player throws himself back onto his shoulders (fig. 2) and immediately folds his legs over himself so that his knees come toward his face (fig. 3).

Keep the legs close together. From the fig. 3 position, push off from the ground forcefully with the arms. Swing the legs directly up and over. Keep your hips high and curl the legs in under yourself to position yourself well for the landing (fig. 4). Land on both feet together and bring your arms forward to help you regain the upright position (fig. 5).

Application in the jogo

This is a floreio, but also a practical solution to returning to your feet with dignity if you find yourself in the fig. 2 position because of a foot sweep. Some players like to jump from fig. 5 to fig. 2 after completing one mola, and repeat the whole cycle a few times to demonstrate their acrobatic ability.

✦

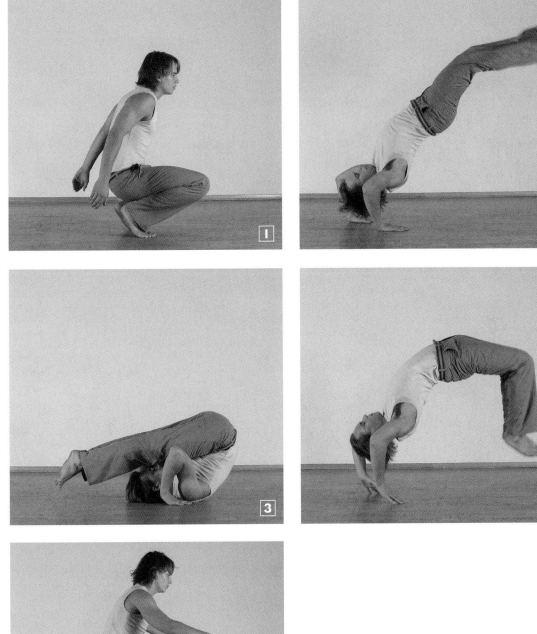
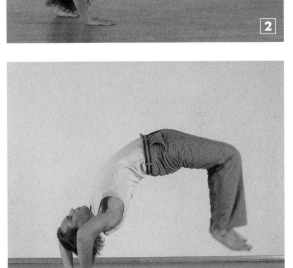
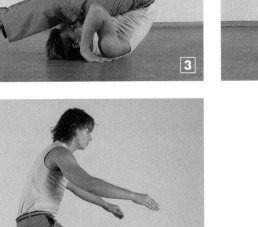

74. Gato

Movement

This movement means "cat." It is similar to a macaco and in gymnastics is called a flic-flac or back handspring.

Pointers

In fig. 1 the player is poised as if he's going to sit down in an invisible chair. Just when he's about to sit in the chair, it's pulled from beneath him. At this point, he throws the arms straight back out behind the head, forcefully, at shoulder width apart, keeping them very straight and locked out at the elbow (fig. 2). It's as if jumping backward into a handstand. The legs flip over the head (fig. 3) and continue, with the feet together, to fig. 4, and finish standing (fig. 5).

Note: When you throw your arms back in gato, follow the trajectory of the movement with your head, keeping the arms straight when you hit the ground with your hands. If you want to stay in the same spot, jump upward as you throw the arms and head back; if you want to gato backward (covering some distance), jump backward and arch as you throw the arms back. The better you can get your ponte and your walkovers, the easier gato will be. Also, practice many macacos first, to get the feel of throwing your body back.

Application in the jogo

This is an excellent movement for mobility at speed within the roda. It is dramatic, acrobatic, and enables you to flic-flac away from techniques or even over the other player's body and movements. Like macaco, gato adds three-dimensionality to your game, and it is a movement used by both Regional players and Angoleiros alike.

❖

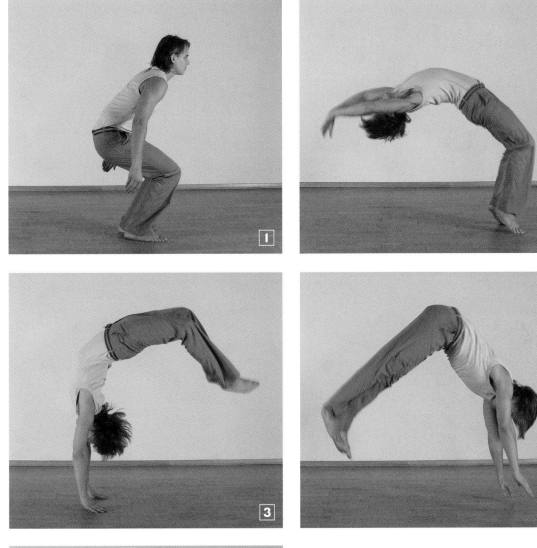

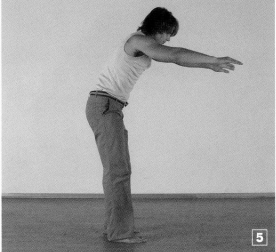

75. Gato
(ON THE FOREARMS)

Movement

This is also a back flic-flac, although here the player catches his body on his forearms rather than his hands.

Pointers

Beginning in cocorinha, the player begins to stand up, and at the point where he is sitting in the aforementioned imaginary chair, he flings his arms backward, simultaneously jumping up and back while arching his spine (fig. 2), reaching for the ground with the side of the hands, the forearms, and elbows (figs. 2 and 3). Notice

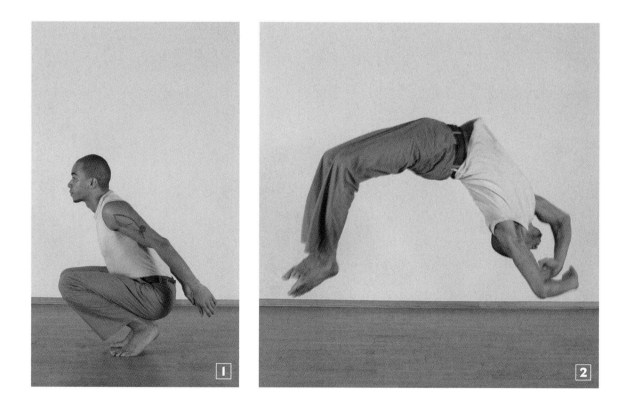

that his head is pulled back, so that when he hits the ground with his forearms, he is looking at the ground, and doesn't hit it with the top of his head (fig. 3). The legs flip straight over and back down to earth (fig. 4).

Application in the jogo

This gato can be used to move in the roda in the same way as the previous technique, with the added demonstration of dexterity shown by playing on the forearms. A lot of players don't practice many movements on their forearms, so playing in this way shows some originality as well.

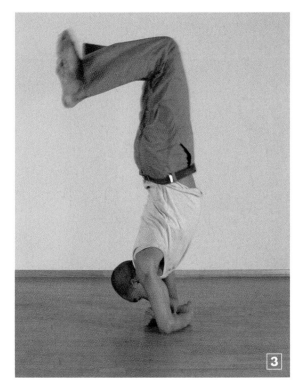

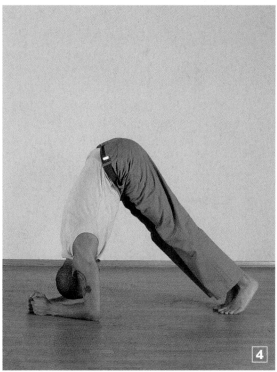

76. Helicóptero

Movement

This is a smooth and surprising technique that can be described as a rotating twist from aú that drives forward a kick in an inverted position.

Pointers

Keep the legs as straight as possible at all stages of the movement. You can almost let the first leg (the leading right foot) hit the floor (fig. 3), keeping it as low as you can get it, as in a normal aú. Keep your eyes on the foot of the first leg. Let the first (right) leg steer the movement as you twist and drive it through figs. 3, 4, and 5. Don't bend the second (left) leg (keep it straight)—it will land on the floor naturally from the momentum of the movement (fig. 6). Rotate through this sequence with enough speed to build momentum to lead through with the first leg and recover an upright position once the second foot has hit the floor.

Application in the jogo

This kick can be used as an attack, and it is very deceptive. It seems at first that the player is moving off in one direction in aú normal, and due to the twist of his body, he kicks back directly in the direction from which he came. In most cases, the player isn't attempting to hammer the other player with the kick of the leading foot, but to weave the movement seamlessly in close proximity to the techniques of the opponent.

✺

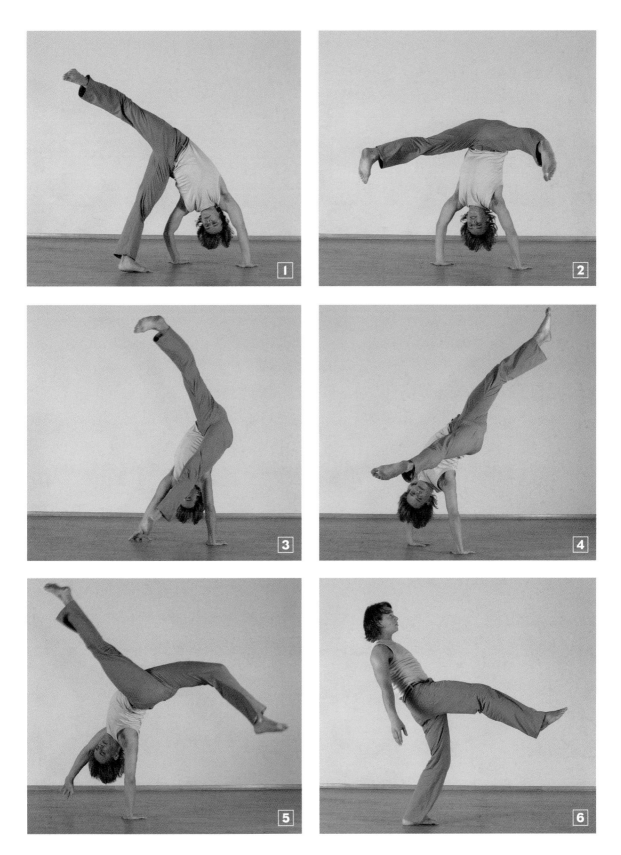

77. Relógio

Movement

This movement is called "clock" because the player's body rotates around on a horizontal circular plane similar to the hands of a clock.

Pointers

To gain enough strength and balance for this movement, try putting both your hands on the floor and placing your elbows in toward your navel. Rest the weight of your body over the elbows and balance your belly on the elbows with the legs off the floor (bent if necessary). To gain the spin, the player shifts the weight onto one elbow and uses the free hand to push around (fig. 1). Gain speed by paddling with the free hand (fig. 2). After gaining sufficient speed, the player raises the free hand and allows the momentum to spin his body on the axis of the elbow (fig. 3). You can finish off by coming out in a queda de rins (fig. 5).

For practice you can place a slippery cloth under your balancing hand to aid the rotation.

Application in the jogo

The relógio is similar to the hand-glide in break-dance. As a floreio it is an impressive technique, though it can also be used as a desequilibrante.

✳

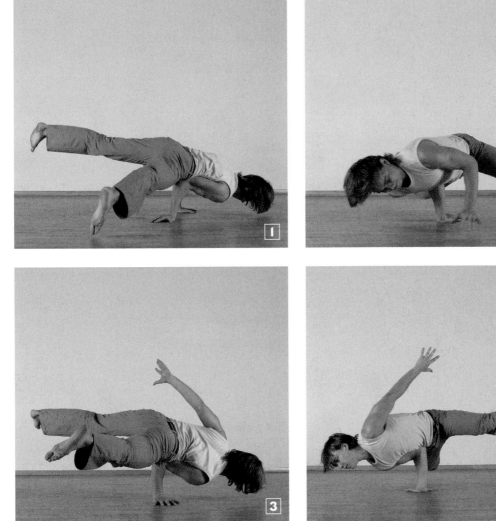

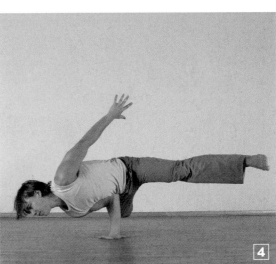

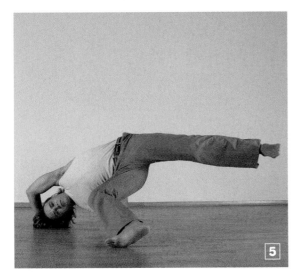

78. Armada Pulada

Movement

This is a jumping armada.

Pointers

Turn as if for an armada (fig. 2). Leap directly upward, getting as much height as possible. Bring the support leg up and tuck it in under the body (fig. 3). A common mistake is to leave the support leg hanging down near the ground, which would make the player vulnerable to rasteira. Land balanced and lightly on two feet, with the kicking (left) leg at the back, where it began (fig. 4).

Note that the leap upward comes first. The leg kicks out for armada once the player is already fully airborne and circling. Some

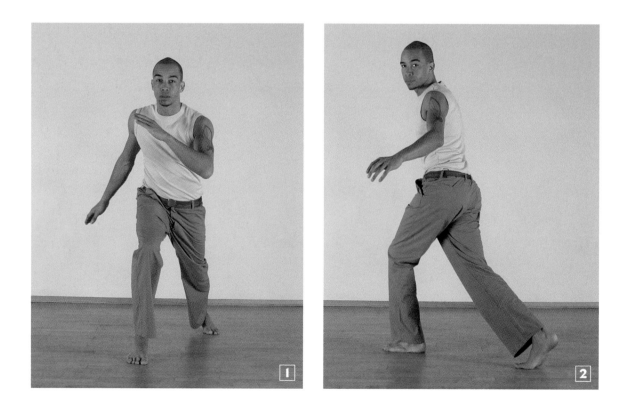

players do a full turn before kicking halfway though the second rotation. You can practice by jumping high and doing a 360° turn in mid-air without a kick (making sure to bring both your knees up and tuck your legs as you do it).

Application in the jogo

This dynamic kick is great for the kind of spectacular games where all the movements are close, well-timed, and done at high speed. It's a kick that packs explosive power and can be aimed at or above the head of the opponent. Armada pulada can also be done in a low game, from a cocorinha. In this case the player leaps straight up from the squat and can land back in a squat again after turning the kick.

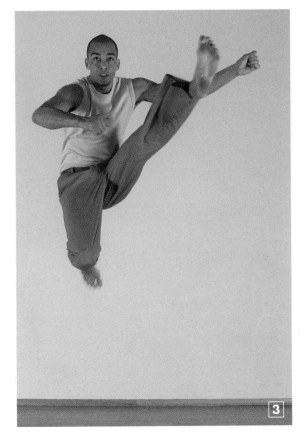

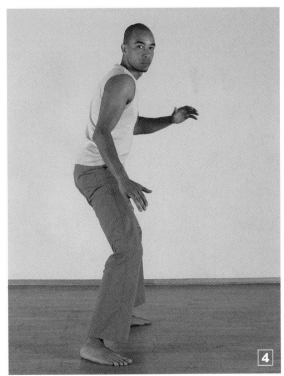

79. Parafuso 1

Movement

Parafuso is a flying kick that "screws" through the air at head height or even over the body of your partner.

Pointers

The player begins as if doing a fast armada with the left leg. In fig. 1 he launches himself into the air, leading with a high left leg. He continues to gain height, following with the right leg (fig. 2) through the same trajectory. The force of his right leg catapults him back over himself (fig. 3). He completes the turn by landing firmly on both feet (fig. 4).

Practice spinning into an armada, until your first leg has reached the front of your body. Jump off the support foot as high as you can.

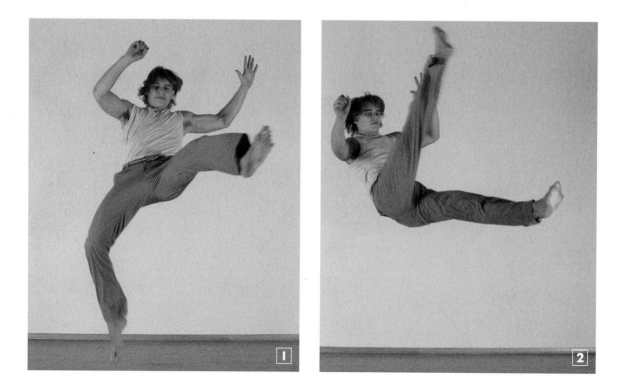

Rotate the hips, as if you are trying to hit an imaginary baseball out of the ball park with the top of your second foot when it reaches the high point of the turn (at the front of your body). Wind around for a 360° rotation and look forward throughout the kick.

Application in the jogo

Parafuso is a technique that enables a capoeirista to play in the air. If the rhythm and tempo speed up, well-timed parafusos are perfect kicks for a dynamic game. Although it is not good form to do high kicks over low movements, flying kicks are another story, and high parafusos can sometimes be seen soaring way over the head of a low-playing capoeirista. Once you have mastered the single parafuso, it is a good idea to try two or three in a row so you are able to fit them into a game that involves multiple turning kicks. With multiple parafusos, the skill is to recover your optimal footing as completely and quickly as you can to launch the next kick.

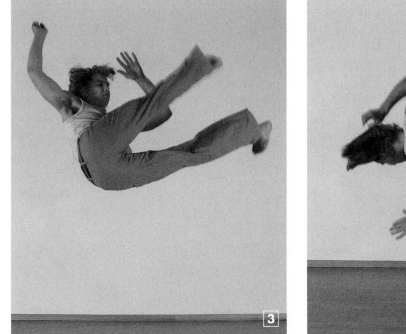

80. Parafuso 2

Movement

This is a different version of essentially the same kick. It builds momentum via the airborne "screw," but delivers the kick with the shin or top of the foot at an angle similar to a martelo de estalo.

Pointers

The initial spin begins here with the lead (left) leg, similar to an armada (figs. 2 and 3). The lead (left) leg should be lifted high to gain height for the aerial screw. As the leg swings around, leap up and forward from the support leg (fig. 4). Continue the turn, committing your entire body: head, shoulders, arms, and waist (fig. 5).

Note that as the kick is aimed (at around head height), the hips are centered onto the target so that the kick is applied with the top of the (right) foot (fig. 6). Don't let your hips sag back and down or you will lose height and also be kicking with the instep rather than top of your foot.

To finish off the movement, the right leg would continue around until it reaches the ground and the player completes the full 360° rotation of her body.

Application in the jogo

Most times parafuso is used in capoeira, it is aimed just above or in front of the opponent rather than intentionally at their head. If you find (as sometimes happens) that you are tending toward doing the same techniques over and over again, it is a good idea to include parafusos for the surprise factor, and to challenge yourself to move out of your own comfort zone once in a while.

❋

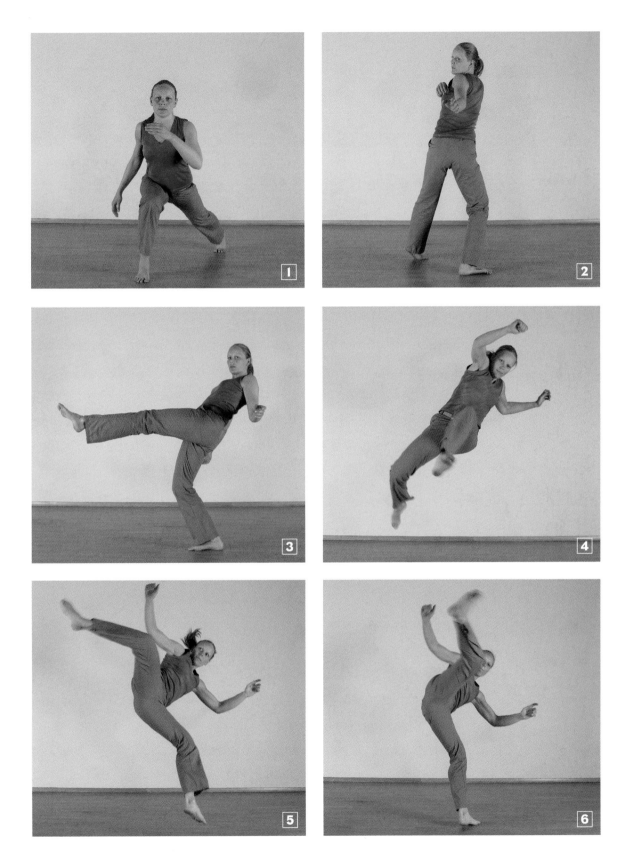

81. Salto Mortal

Movement

This is an aerial back somersault done from a standing start without a run up (although some players do salto mortal with a run up).

Pointers

Don't look at the ground before you begin this movement. Look directly ahead of yourself and just higher than your own eye level. Keep this visual focus for as long as possible through the initial vertical jump phase of the movement.

Take your arms back and bend your legs in preparation for the jump (fig. 1). When you bend your knees you can go quite low, though no deeper than a 90° angle. As strongly as you can, raise your arms straight upward to propel yourself as high as possible for the jump. This is a vertical jump in an upward rather than backward direction.

At the very peak of this upward vertical jump, tuck the knees in (keeping your legs close together) for the roll-over. As you tuck your knees, bring them toward your chest while simultaneously bringing your arms back in toward your legs. Some people grab their knees or the back of their thighs at this stage, or you can have your arms in on either side of your legs as in the pictures (figs. 3 and 4).

Note: Don't tuck the legs in too early. Wait until the upward jump has reached its top position, aided by the upward swing of your arms. When full height is achieved, only then roll over with the tuck (thus ensuring you gain enough height for the roll).

When you land, try to land on the whole flat sole of the foot, and not the heel or the toes alone (figs. 5 and 6). Recover the upright

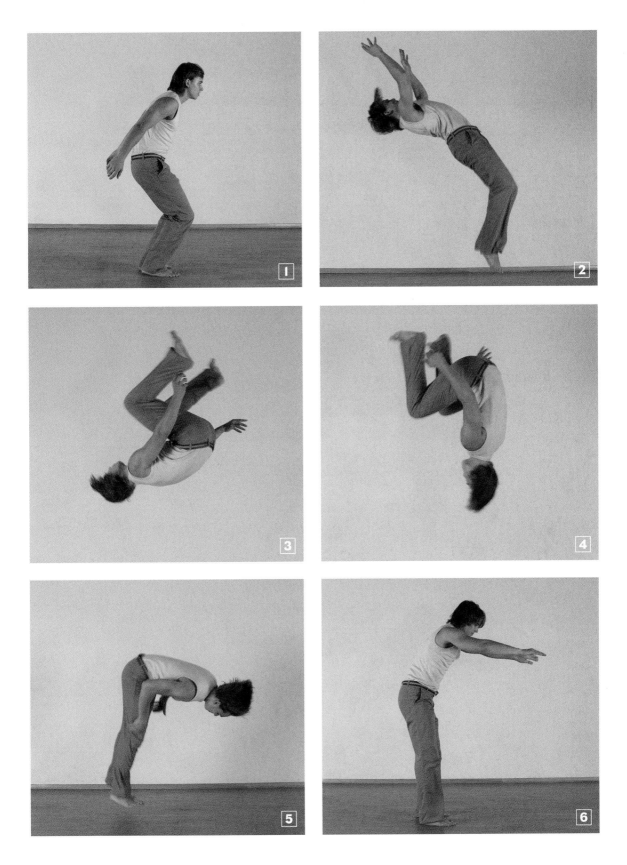

position as quickly as possible so that you're ready to resume the game.

Note: If you don't do back flips off a diving board or on a trampoline, to practice salto mortal initially, it is a good idea to use an experienced spotter who knows the movement well and can help with your performance. Acrobatic and gymnastic coaches as well as capoeiristas who are experienced in saltos may all be useful in this regard.

Application in the jogo

Sometimes capoeira "traditionalists" criticize the use of salto mortal in the jogo, saying that it reduces capoeira to the level of "mere acrobatics" or even worse, "a circus performance." Yet the historical record shows that capoeira has always been an acrobatic art form, involving leaps and daring somersaults. Representatives from the Congo in Brazil, demonstrating their fighting prowess in the seventeenth century, did all sorts of somersaults.

Mestre Decânio in his book, *Herança de Bimba*, related that Mestre Bentinho, an African-born capoeira player in Salvador (of the late nineteenth and early twentieth centuries), could do "a salto mortal inside the mouth of a big box of onions." The knowledgeable old master, Tiburcinho, relayed that "Besouro Mangangá was able to flip backwards and land in his sandals!" This deed, according to Decânio, wasn't rare among the old capoeiristas, and he regretted that these kinds of abilities were seldom seen anymore.

The application of salto mortal in the jogo de capoeira has two parts—the first being for shows and performances, and the second for the game. Saltos are popular with audiences who know little of capoeira because they are spectacular. Therefore there is a place for saltos to impress audiences with capoeira's potential and versatility.

However, capoeira that consists only of flips and saltos is boring. Many circus acrobats and even relatively modest gymnasts can do better somersaults than the vast majority of capoeiristas, so the position of salto mortal in capoeira is always going to be limited. Otherwise circus acrobats would be considered capoeira masters, which clearly they are not.

This leaves the second function of the salto, as a movement to be played within the game itself. It is always better to connect it to the flow of the action, to be done while playing at close range with a partner. Two players with no connection to each other flipping around in different areas of a massive roda are not really doing capoeira. But when a player can throw a salto strategically, while reacting to an opponent, it is a very skillful movement that adds to rather than detracts from the jogo de capoeira.

❖

Partner Sequences

82. Chapéu de Couro — Esquiva Lateral

Movement

The attacking player here has his right hand on the floor and right leg extended in negativa (fig. 1). He uses chapéu de couro to jump over an esquiva lateral.

Pointers

To begin the movement, hop forcefully off the left foot while at the same time swinging the right leg both upward and forward over or toward the target, depending on what you want to do. In the photo, the player's intention is to swing over his partner. Everything should be thrown in the same direction, the first (right) leg, the left arm, and also the hips. As with macaco, it is vital to swing the hips up to gain height and momentum. The second leg follows through the same trajectory as the lead leg. To come out of the movement, land on the far side of the defender's head and rolé.

Application in the jogo

This is a kick or a floreio, useful for kicking upward at or over a target from the ground.

✳

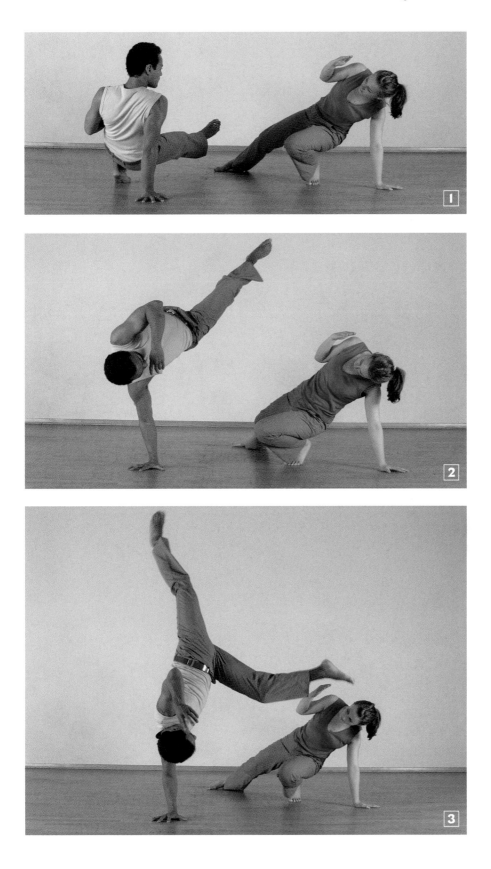

83. Bênção — Esquiva

Movement

The attacker kicks with bênção, and the defending player leans back exaggeratedly from the waist.

Pointers

Timing is vital here, as the player must lean back in time and far enough to escape the kick. It may be necessary to raise the heels to gain enough backward lean to make this an effective esquiva.

Application in the jogo

This is a stylish esquiva, although it contains inherent risks, the main one being that the defending player remains in a precarious and vulnerable position even though he or she is doing an esquiva. This esquiva can be converted into a walkover, or a counterattack, by dropping low for a queda de rins and rasteira or a negativa de solo. It would be good to say that the esquiva would convert into a gato with a kick under the attacker's chin on the way over, but this would be getting carried away.

·❋·

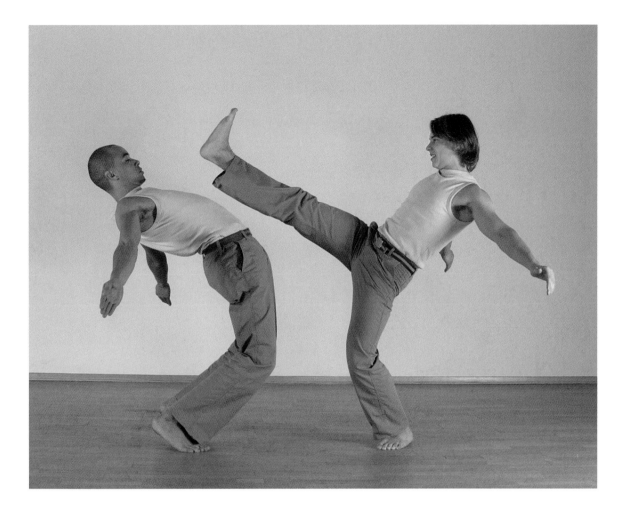

84. Cabeçada—Aú Normal

Movement

This technique is sometimes called *arpão de cabeça* and is a head-butt. Head-butts, along with rasteiras (foot sweeps), were the main fighting movements of the capoeirista in nineteenth-century Brazil and earlier. The picture here depicts a basic cabeçada to counter an aú normal. In fig. 1, the player positions himself as soon as he sees his opponent go for the aú normal. By pulling the arms back (fig. 2), he propels his head at the other player's belly.

Pointers

Position your weight directly over the front thigh. If you lunge too far forward you will not have stable balance. Use the backward swing of the two arms and the power of the push forward off your back foot to accelerate your head directly at the target. Some beginners move slightly backward or to the side with their head before the direct cabeçada. This wastes time and dissipates the power of the cabeçada. The head should move toward the target by the most direct route.

Application in the jogo

It is often only necessary to show a cabeçada. Just make contact with the intended target area; do not feel that you have to power your opponent off balance at every opportunity. Part of the strategy of the jogo de capoeira is to find the openings in your partner's game and show what you could have done without actually going ahead and doing it. Cabeçada is useful if the opponent is very focused on your feet and kicks, and not paying attention to your head.

Note that the player doing aú normal might kick directly downward onto the back of the player doing cabeçada with an aú batendo
counterattack.

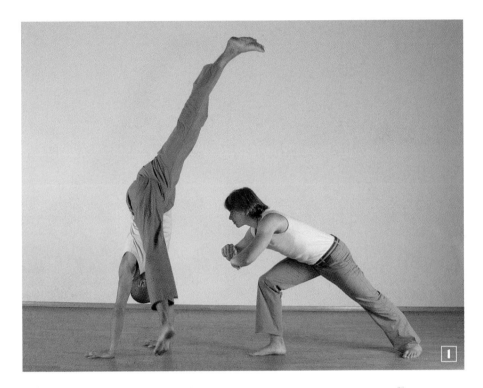

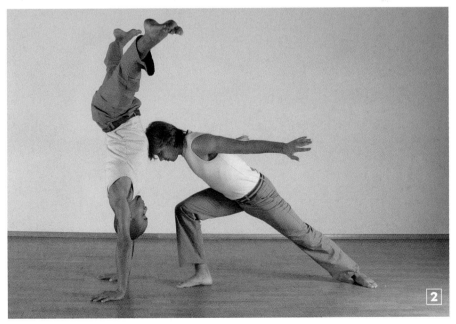

85. Bênção—Esquiva para Trás

Movement

The bênção kick is sometimes called *chapa de frente*. It is a direct front kick, delivered by bringing the knee high, straightening the leg, and pushing forward with the hip. The sole of the kicking foot hits the target. The kick can be aimed at any point between the groin and the head. In Capoeira Angola, where it is called *chapa de frente no peito*, this movement tends to be kicked at around waist height.

The esquiva here, para trás, means an "escape backward." The player steps and leans back from the waist to get out of range of the kicking foot. He is sideways to the other player, but as always, keeps his partner in his sight. Don't esquiva until the last moment, just before the kicking foot is about to make contact with your body.

Pointers

When you kick with bênção, keep the heel of the supporting foot firmly on the floor—don't rise onto your toes. Pull the toes of the kicking foot back so the kick is done with the heel end of the sole for extra power. (If you extend the foot and kick with the ball it would be a ponteira, not a bênção.) The power of bênção comes from the push forward with the hips, so focus on bringing the knee up before your kick and push hard as you extend the leg. Make sure of your distance from your partner when you do bênção. If you are too close you may become entangled and thrown off balance.

The arms are extended at the sides of the player executing the kick. This keeps the body in balance and fits with capoeira's style, which generally disguises obvious fighting stances.

Application in the jogo

It is possible to do this with a lot of speed, so take it easy and remember to play to the rhythm of the music. Fast kicks like this are relatively easy to catch an opponent with, so try to use them with some panache—for example, timing it to catch the other player completely by surprise as they come out of a technique. Doing ginga and kicking out with random bênçãos to no purpose is not the most effective use of the kick.

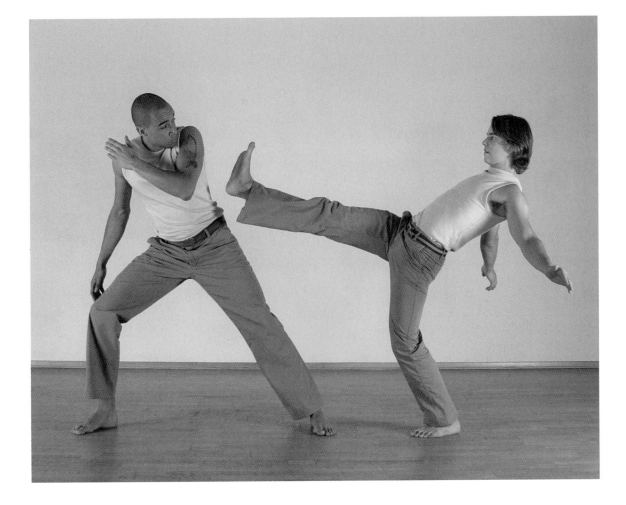

86. Meia Lua de Compasso — Esquiva Lateral

Movement

Here is another type of esquiva to avoid many types of turning and spinning kicks—in this case, meia lua de compasso. In the photograph, we see that the first player has spun around with a swinging meia lua de compasso, a heel kick. The defender has bent his right leg and used his right hand on the ground for stability, while lowering his hips and defending his face with the left hand.

Pointers

Both players are watching each other closely. The defending player esquivas low enough to avoid the kick. Make sure you esquiva to escape kicks completely, as the kicker shouldn't have to pull or heighten his or her kicks to avoid kicking you. It is each player's task to avoid being kicked to the best of their ability.

Application in the jogo

Esquiva lateral is common in the game of capoeira. It can easily convert into an aú, a negativa lateral, a rolé, an aú quebrado, or a change of direction into a negativa normal followed by chapéu de couro or S-dobrado. Use esquiva lateral to defend against martelo, martelo giratório, armada, queixada, meia lua de frente, etc.

❖

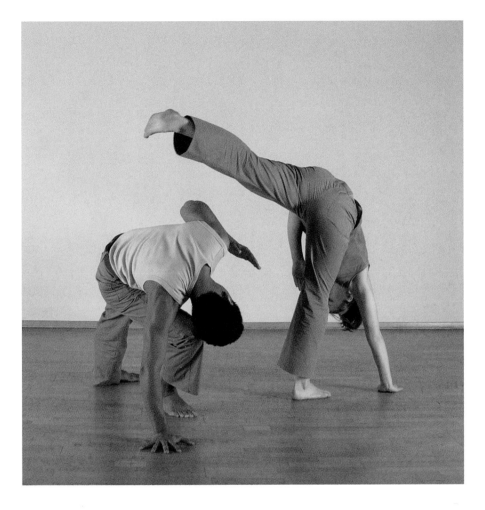

87. Cabeçada (Angola style) — Aú Normal

Movement

This is cabeçada, though here it's called cabeçada (Angola) simply to distinguish it from the first type of cabeçada (No. 84). In this movement the player begins in cocorinha, and then he shoots his body forward to hit his opponent's exposed chest with the top of his head (figs. 2 and 3).

Pointers

In fig. 2, the player doesn't come off the ground. From cocorinha (fig. 1) he keeps his feet where they are but strikes forward with the top of his head. Try to ensure that it is your body shooting forward from the feet and then being supported on the hands, rather than the common mistake of dropping the hands early and shooting the feet backward (which takes you in the opposite direction you want to go).

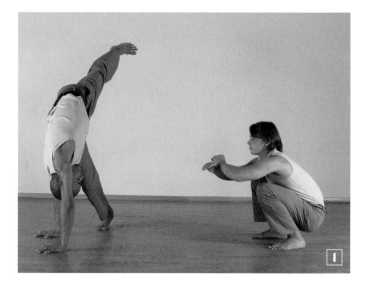

Do not sag at the waist as you do this movement. A sagging waist will shorten the length of the movement and decrease its power. In fig. 3 the player launches himself at his target like a missile. Remember to hit the target with the top of your head and angle the cabeçada from the ground upward to gain maximum power.

Application in the jogo

The position in fig. 3 enables you to launch a cabeçada from a distance. This type of head-butt doesn't only work from cocorinha; it will work just as effectively from ginga and other positions. It can be done to attack under a movement, such as going for the ribs after a player has just done a rabo de arraia. To commit yourself to this movement takes some confidence, so make sure that you are certain of the timing and the target (as you don't want to launch yourself head-first at your opponent's rear end instead of their ribs or chest).

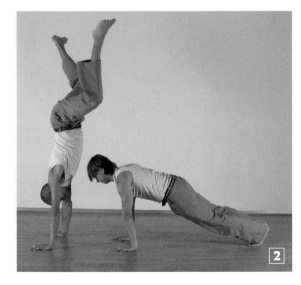 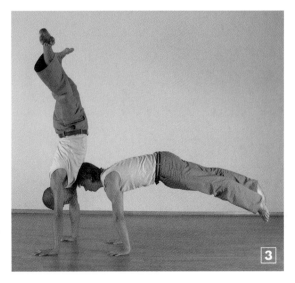

88. Armada— Resistençia

Movement

This short sequence shows the way the resistençia technique can be used to duck in under a kick (in this case, armada) and position the defender well to counterattack the opposing player.

Pointers

When practicing esquivas in sequence with a partner, don't drop until the last moment. Make sure that the resistençia is a response to the kick. Work on understanding your partner's direction by reading clues in their movements in advance of attacks. When you drop into the resistençia, have the hand up on the side from which the attack is coming for extra defense of your face. Sink right down on your haunches and put one hand on the floor to differentiate this technique from Nos. 9 (fig. 1) and 10.

Application in the jogo

This is a way of evading a kick without moving out of range of the other player. Look at the player squatting in resistençia and try to imagine how many techniques he is now in a position to counter with: tesoura, cabeçada, chapa de costas, alavanca, rasteira, negativa de solo as a sweep. These are just a few of the counterattacks that could be delivered quickly from the defender's position in fig. 3.

※

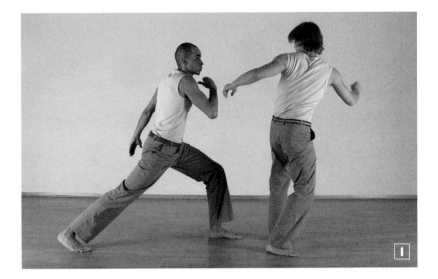

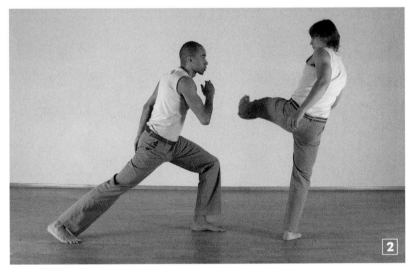

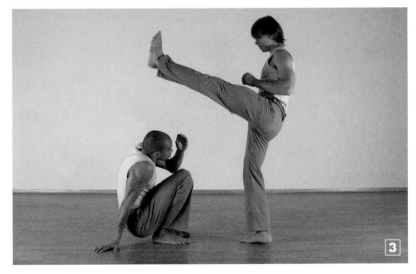

89. Armada — Parafuso

Movement

This sequence shows the player closely following an armada with a parafuso. In fig. 1, the player on the left has just done an armada, beneath which the player on the right has done an esquiva to position himself for a follow-up parafuso.

Pointers

To practice this sequence, begin close to a partner. Drill the sequence of ducking under the armada with esquiva (fig. 1) and follow by twisting around and throwing up the back (left) leg so that it leads into the jump (fig. 2). Take the leading leg as high as possible. In figs. 3 and 4 the player doing the parafuso has both legs high. In fig. 5 he has rotated his hips and slapped over the right leg for the parafuso.

Application in the jogo

This is used both as a floreio and a kick. There isn't a great deal to do to counter a leaping parafuso in progress other than aim for a perfectly timed sweep when the player lands. Parafuso is an exciting and skillful maneuver, testing a player's timing and athleticism.

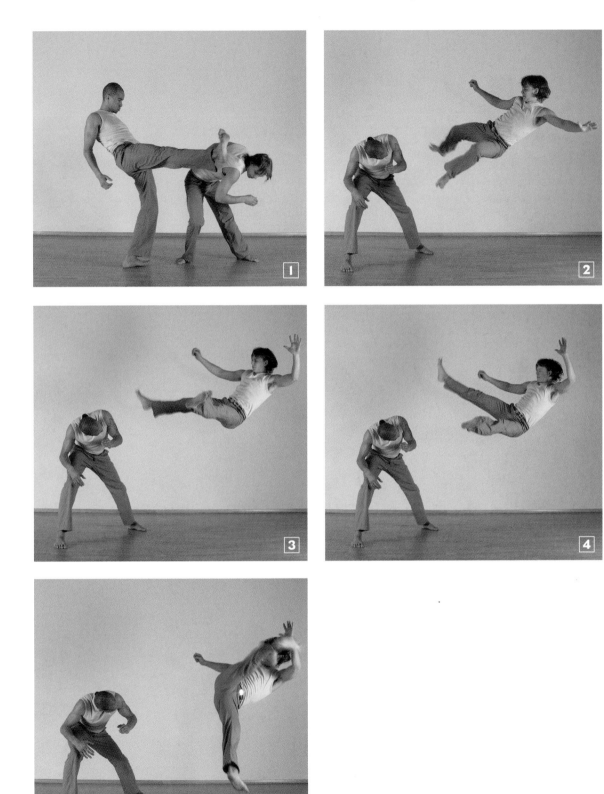

90. Meia Lua de Compasso — Esquiva to Ponte (Bridge Walkover)

Movement

The first player directs a meia lua de compasso at his partner. The second player brings her arms and hands up in front of her face, pushes her hips well forward, and esquivas back in a low "limbo dancing" posture. In fig. 2 she lets herself fall back, shooting both arms directly out beyond her head to catch her fall. In fig. 3, having pushed up into a bridge, she does a walkover to come out of the movement.

Pointers

For the limbo position of the esquiva, make sure you control your weight well by clenching your buttocks and using the back of the thighs to support your body weight. The knees are plunged forward and low to the ground.

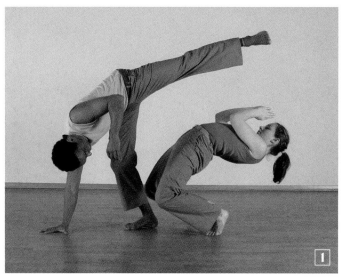

Note: In fig. 2, when the defending player shoots her arms rapidly out toward the floor, she keeps her chin tucked in and her head forward so that she doesn't hit her head against the floor. For pointers on the walkover (fig. 3), see No. 91 below.

Application in the jogo

The ability to slip and slide at a low angle, horizontal to the floor, is one of the defining characteristics of capoeira. This way of playing adds "three-dimensionality" to your game. It enables you to esquiva instantaneously regardless of which angle you are at to your partner when attacked. The more slippery your esquivas are, the better.

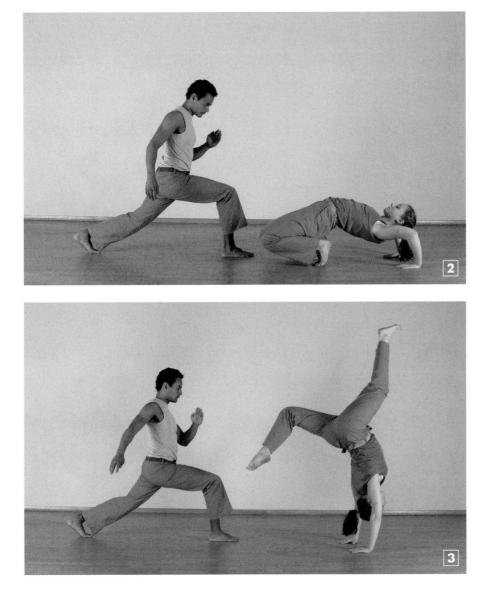

91. Ponte Walkover: Breaking It Down

Movement

Here the player begins in a ponte, raises one leg, pushes off with the other, and walks straight over herself.

Pointers

If she began in the fig. 2 position from No. 90, she would raise her hips, straighten her arms, and push up into the bridge ponte shown here in fig. 1. From this foundation, she kicks up forcefully with her (left) leg, while pushing off with her right (fig. 2). This creates momentum for the walkover (fig. 3). She lands on the (left) leg (fig. 4) and stands up again.

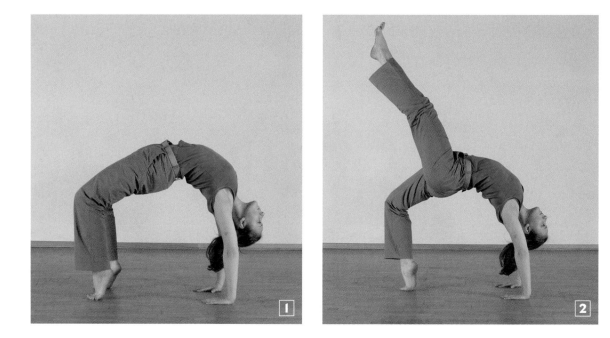

Application in the jogo

There are many techniques in capoeira that circle in a horizontal plane (such as the kicking leg in armada and rabo de arraia, the whole body in relógio, etc.). There are also techniques which circle at a semi-horizontal or semi-vertical angle, such as chapéu de couro, parafuso, and so on.

To gain the full spectrum of techniques, do the circles that loop over themselves head over heels or vice versa, such as gato, macaco, salto mortal, aú espinha, and the ponte with a walkover. These movements increase versatility and the range of possibilities open to you in the roda.

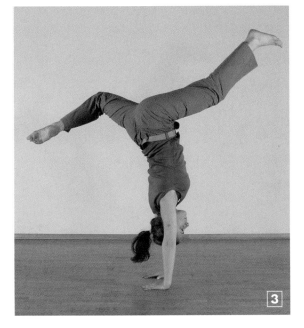

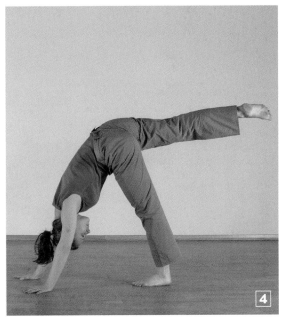

92. Vingativa

Movement

This is an unambiguous desequilibrante. The player brings his or her whole extended leg up behind the two feet of the opponent. With a quick pivot of the torso and the assistance of the right arm (or elbow for a more vicious technique), the player levers the opponent over the leg (fig. 2).

Pointers

Make sure that the lever leg comes up behind both the opponent's feet. Try to work on a smooth motion that sweeps and "bumps" the lever leg forward simultaneously to knock the opponent back with your arm in the center of their chest.

Application in the jogo

The skill of doing this movement without turning the game into a wrestling match is in positioning yourself perfectly to take your partner by surprise. This can be achieved by coming in from the side just after the partner has completed a technique and is still unsteady on his feet.

Another way is to distract your partner with a harmless-looking movement like corta capim, and with the final swing bring the rotating leg up to the side and then back behind the opponent's legs for a rapidly delivered vingativa.

A well-timed maneuver that unbalances is superior to one that relies on brute force (not timing) to take the opponent down.

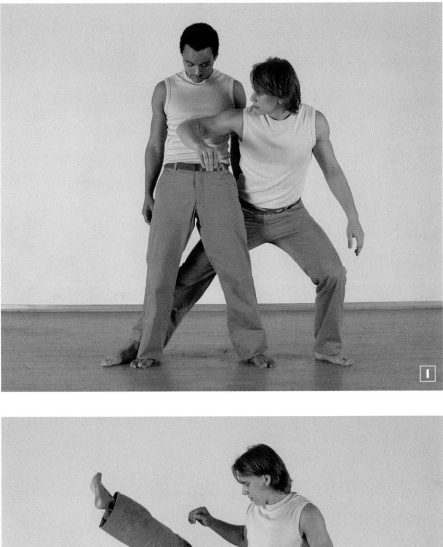

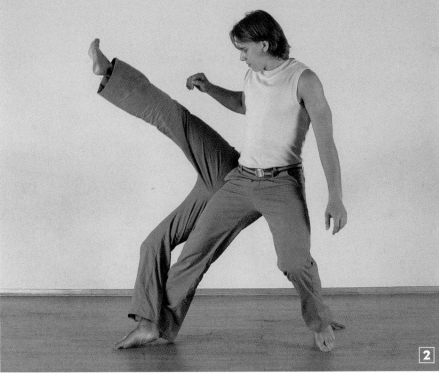

93. Tesoura 1

Movement

This technique is sometimes called *tesoura de costas*. Tesoura translates to "scissors" and is another desequilibrante—a movement that unbalances the other player.

Pointers

The player doing the tesoura jumps at his opponent, entrapping his body within two pivoting legs, twisting forcefully at the waist, so that the feet of the defender are pulled out from underneath him in one direction, and his torso is forced backward in the other. It isn't necessary to tesoura as high as the players in the photograph, though try to get the lower tesoura leg completely behind both of the opponent's legs. The upper tesoura leg should be across their body at any point between their knees and their chest.

Note: If the tesoura is too low, you will get no leverage on your opponent's limbs and you will end up lying on the floor yourself, dragging on their ankles. If a tesoura doesn't work immediately, extract yourself from it immediately and don't keep "flogging a dead horse," as the saying goes.

Application within the jogo

Given good timing, the tesoura can be done quite lightly. It doesn't have to be a full-blown body slam. It's a fun technique to do against a player you know—one who knows how to fall and won't take it the wrong way if you commit yourself to taking them down. Be aware that this move can be dangerous. If the other player is whipped over too quickly, he can bang the back of his head on the floor. Do this movement only with people who have experience in capoeira and know how to fall.

It's not a good idea to go into a roda full of strangers and utilize a tesoura on players who are unknown to you. This applies to any movement that requires contact directly with your partner with the intention of putting them down, such as vingativa, tesoura, rasteira, etc. Watch a roda and get a feel of its atmosphere before playing yourself.

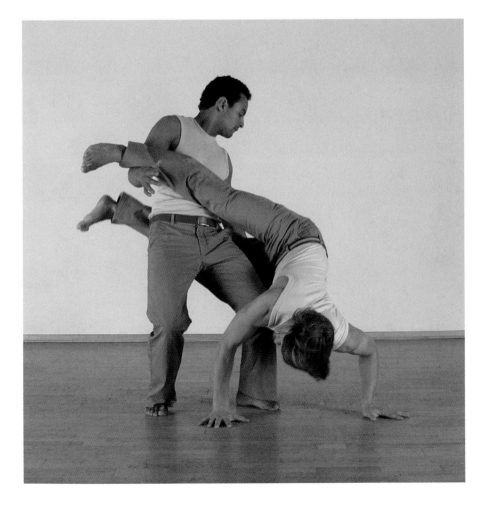

94. Tesoura 2

Movement

This is also a scissor movement. This time you lever with the front thigh of your top leg. In the photo the player has applied the lever against the whole body of his opponent. He could also have applied the tesoura 2 with his right (top) thigh pushing down just above the knee(s) of his opponent.

Pointers

Lever forward and downward with the top leg, focusing on pushing the opponent to the ground with your thigh.

Application in the jogo

This takedown should be done quickly and unexpectedly. The same applies to No. 93. Tesouras are techniques that work well at the moment a player has just completed a kick such as armada, before he or she has regained total equilibrium and orientation.

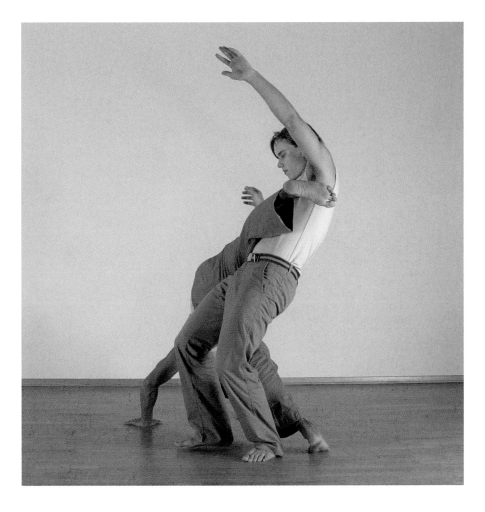

95. Tesoura—Aú Compasso

Movement

This kind of tesoura is a scissors movement that slides in toward your partner along the ground. The aú compasso is an effective escape from this trapping movement.

Pointers

The player can slide toward his or her partner from some distance away. Keep the tesoura low, so that you are horizontal with the ground, though only your hands and feet touch the ground. Do not have your legs spread wide open in tesoura, but have the upper leg folded over the lower one to protect your groin. Look over your shoulder at your target. To move along the ground, shuffle your hands rapidly and swivel the waist and torso forcefully to slide smoothly toward your partner.

Note: It sometimes helps to have the side of your feet rather than toes down during tesoura, especially if you have rubber-soled shoes that stick on the ground.

Application in the jogo

If the player doesn't evade this technique quickly enough, pivot your body and take them down with a regular tesoura. As you see, the player here escapes in figs. 2 and 3 by doing an aú compasso out to the blind side of the player sliding in with tesoura. It is important that she moves to the blind side, behind his back, as many players slide in with tesoura with the intention of a follow-up technique such as cabeçada or chapa no chão. The closed aú compasso is further protection against this.

✦

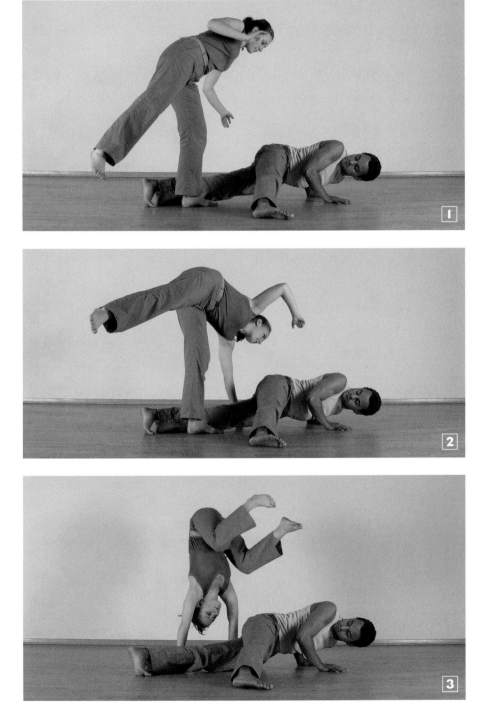

96. Tesoura— Aú Normal

Movement

This is the same sequence as No. 95, with the exception that the defending player escapes with aú normal instead of aú compasso.

Pointers

The same points apply here as for the previous sequence. Sometimes you get a feeling for your opponent's intentions. If you feel confident that they are unlikely to counter-move, it is feasible to escape this tesoura with a wide-open aú normal.

Application in the jogo

These tesoura and escape techniques have similar uses, although the open aú normal can be converted into pião de mão, espinha, and even aú batendo if it seems that the player doing the tesoura is moving for a counter.

✳

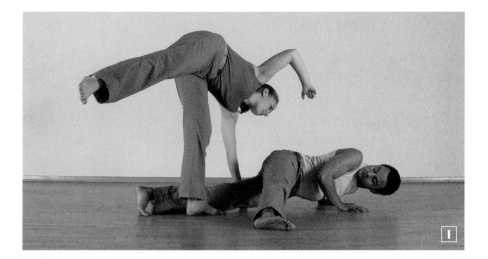

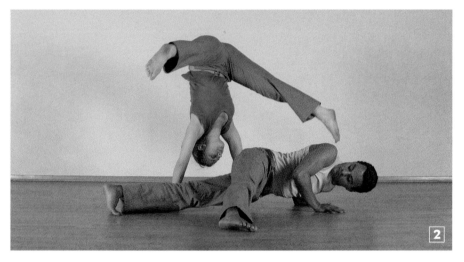

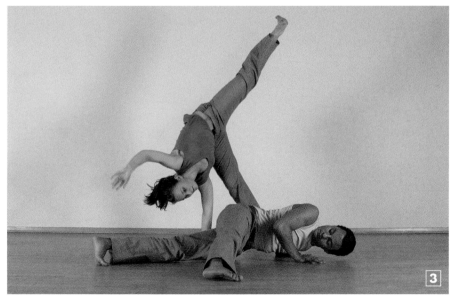

97. Aú Batendo — Rolé

Movement

This kicks down from above during an aú normal.

Pointers

When you do aú batendo, kick with the top of the foot you take off with (the leading leg) in the aú. If you aú to your left, your left hand goes to the ground first, and you would batendo with your right foot. In this picture, the player has done the aú to her right, so she kicks with her left foot.

Note: Have the second leg back as far as you need to get a good counterbalance as you are kicking. Having done batendo, pull the kicking foot back up and exit the aú in the regular way.

Application in the jogo

Even though a player's back is often not a great target for kicks, because it's a closed part of their body anyway, the aú batendo is an exception. It can be done toward a player's head or back if they come in close with a rolé, a cabeçada, or other suspicious intention.

❂

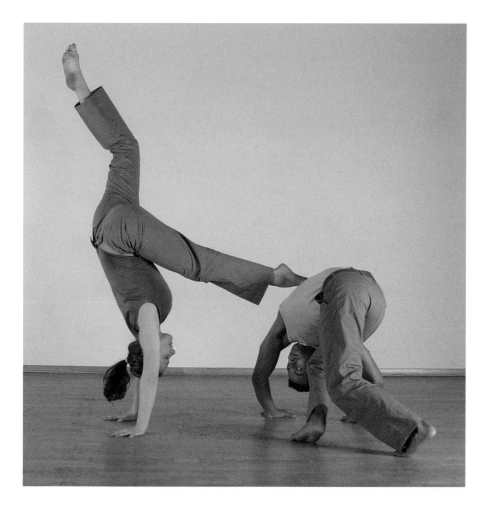

98. Meia Lua de Compasso — Esquiva Lateral — Aú Quebrado

Movement

The second player, having done an esquiva lateral under a meia lua de compasso, immediately counterattacks with an aú quebrado.

Pointers

The defending player does the aú quebrado without raising his right hand from the ground. He pushes up off his right foot and simultaneously kicks forward and down with his left leg, toward the player who just did the meia lua de compasso.

Application in the jogo

The aú quebrado is an attack movement that flows seamlessly from defensive movements. It is a useful kick for following through from esquivas in this way.

❋

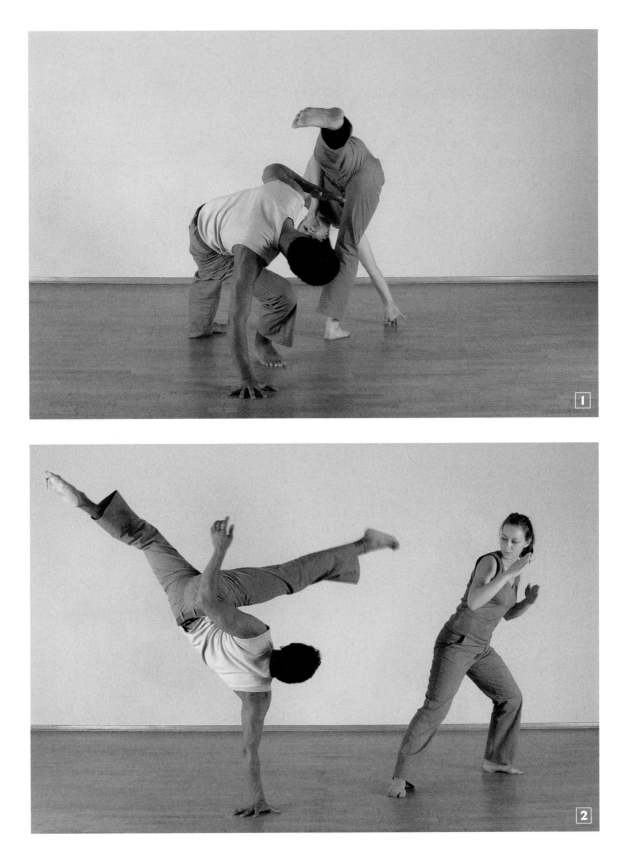

99. Martelo de Estalo—Aú Normal

Movements

The first player does a martelo (hammer kick), while the second player esquivas straight into an aú normal.

Pointers

Esquiva in response to the martelo, not before. Practice aiming the martelo at different heights: the head, the shoulder, and the ribs. When you do your aú, try circling in on your partner, so you don't aú far away from them (figs. 4 and 5).

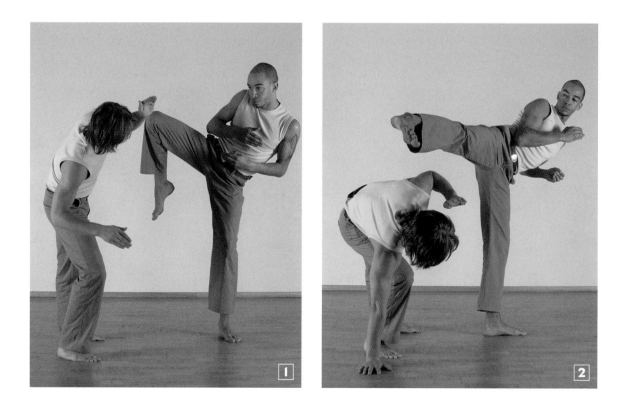

Application in the jogo

It is good practice to follow an esquiva with another technique, such as the aú normal. The capoeira game consists of many linked movements. See what other techniques might link here. The player who has completed the martelo might shoot straight forward to deliver a cabeçada against the open aú normal.

The martelo player (in fig. 4) still has most of the weight on his front (left) foot. The aú player could drop straight down into queda de rins with his left elbow into his waist, and sweep the front foot with a rasteira.

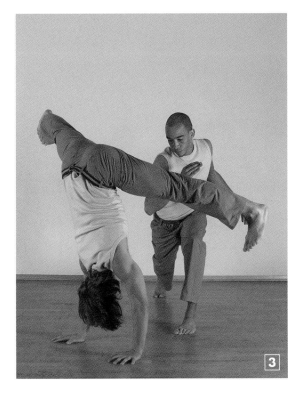
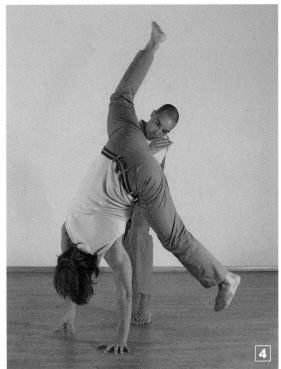

100. Queixada— Armada—Meia Lua de Compasso

Movements

This is a sequence of six kicks that all follow one from another. It is excellent training for close-proximity turning kicks and esquivas with a partner.

Description

Fig. 1: The first player steps forward and puts her weight on her left foot in preparation for the queixada. Her partner begins to lean back in a basic esquiva.

Fig. 2: The first player kicks around with her left leg for queixada, and her partner bends further to esquiva under the kick.

Fig. 3: The first player has taken her left leg to the back and leans over it. The second player slides forward, shifting his weight to his front (right) foot in preparation for his queixada.

Fig. 4: The second player kicks his (right front leg) queixada around over the torso of his partner, who esquivas slightly lower.

Fig. 5: The first player pivots on her feet and looks over her left shoulder in preparation for an armada, which she will deliver with her rear (left) leg. The second player has taken his right leg to the back and begins his esquiva.

Fig. 6: The first player rotates fully to kick over her partner with her (left) leg. He esquivas by leaning back over his right leg.

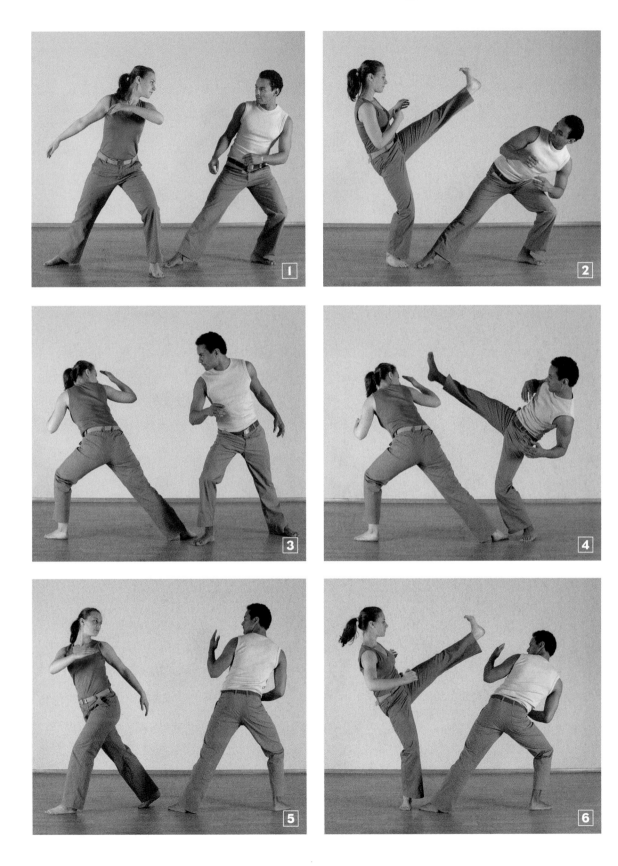

Fig. 7: The second player swivels slightly on his feet and turns to look over his right shoulder in preparation for his armada. The first player begins her esquiva by leaning over her back left leg.

Fig. 8: The second player rotates fully and kicks his armada directly over the body of the first player with his right leg (which he will take to the back again to prepare for the meia lua de compasso).

Fig. 9: At this point both players have now done one queixada and one armada each. They both drop and do a meia lua de compasso, the first player with her left leg, the second with his right. The first player has kicked off before Player 2, so she waits in position as his leg follows a split second behind her.

Note: If the leading player completes her kick early and begins to come up while Player 2's kick is still swinging toward her, she could get kicked in the face. It is important that she wait for fig. 10 to happen before beginning to come out of the kick.

Fig. 10: Player 2 has caught up so that they both turn the kick at the top of the movement simultaneously, their legs virtually touching but not crashing. From this point they would bring the kicking foot to the back as they stand up into fig. 11.

Note: For a full explanation of meia lua de compasso, see No. 32.

Fig. 11: Both players have come up out of the meia lua de compasso. The first player has taken her left leg to the back, and the second player has taken his right leg to the back. At this point they would repeat the sequence of six total kicks, only this time in the opposite direction.

Pointers

When doing the kicks the other way after the first set of six, there is no need to ginga between sets, as your feet are already in position to begin the queixadas in the other direction. Do the whole cycle at

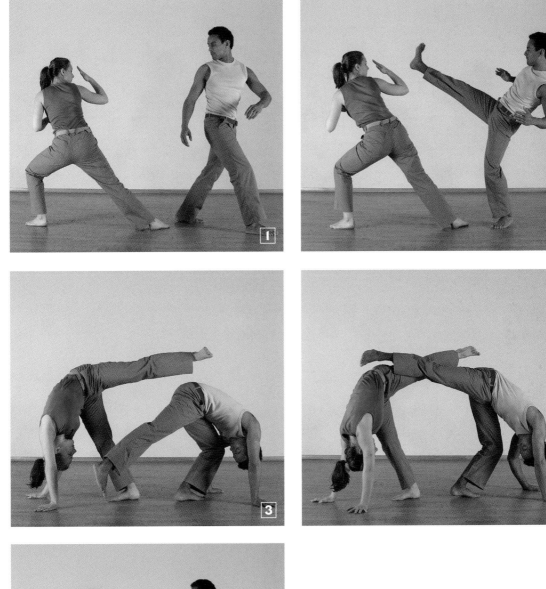

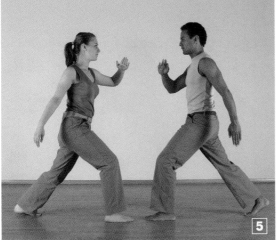

least four times, with Player 1 leading the kicks in both directions, and then Player 2 leading the kicks in both directions.

All the kicks are done with straight legs. The support leg can be slightly bent at the knee, but the kicking leg should be straight. Do this sequence slowly at first, and then speed up, but never go so fast that you are out of control of your movements. Speed will come; quality of the techniques is more important to begin with.

Application in the jogo

The jogo de capoeira is improvised and doesn't follow set sequences. Practicing set sequences prepares you to move with agility and good timing. The coordination required to move constantly at close range during this sequence will improve your ability to do the same thing in the roda.

❂

PART TWO

100 Exercises

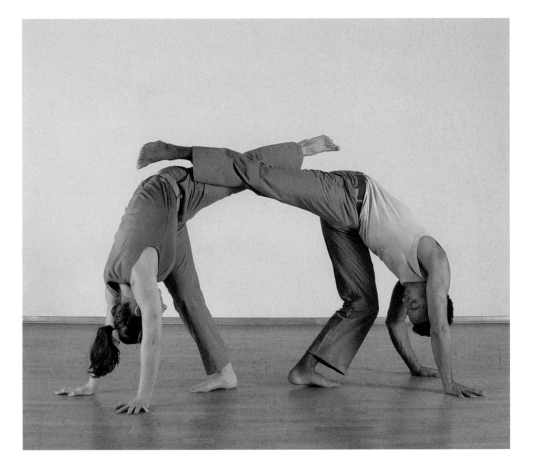

100 Capoeira Exercises, Sequences, and Games to improve your skills and conditioning

General Comments on the Routines

These exercises, games, and sequences are given to help readers train many of the movements shown in this book. They are not laid down as a course to be followed in chronological order, but rather as ideas to try out as and when you feel like it. These activities will keep training varied and cover a wide range of different techniques. Many of the routines can be added to each other to make longer sequences, or sequences that join ground movements with more upright kicks. All of the sequences and exercises have been tried and tested in capoeira classes and workshops with good results.

Some of the exercises are called "focus games." These are games that allow only certain capoeira movements, a restricted roda size, a particular way of playing or such. These encourage a student to focus on a particular aspect of play and help to increase skill in that special area.

Other routines will build conditioning and strength. These set sequences force the body to adapt to performing physically demanding capoeira movements. These movements are not necessarily demanding in terms of skill level, but repeated practice will tax the muscles and cardio-vascular system, and build all-around strength and flexibility.

Many sequences challenge the player to practice balance, jumping kicks, defensive techniques, and linked movements that enhance "flow" in the game and fluidity in the body.

Left and Right

All exercises will be 100% more effective if they are practiced in both directions. If, for example, you are training a meia lua de compasso to the right, it is vital that you also train it to the left. Never train a movement only to one side because that is your good side. (Most people have a good side and a weaker side, even if this only becomes obvious when doing certain techniques.) It is common for beginners to do aú normal without difficulty in one direction, but to get shaky when trying it the other way. This will pass, so persevere.

If you find that you are weak on one side—for example, when doing an aú to the left—don't give up and get into a "that's my bad side, I don't do that side" mentality. On the contrary, it's beneficial to train the movement 50% **more often** to the weak side to make up the balance. For every 10 aús to the right, do 15 to the left to bring this side up to speed. You will be amazed at the improvement in overall coordination, which creates benefits beyond the capoeira roda.

In partner routines, both players should always do techniques to both sides, whether the instruction involves left and right or East and West. If your partner continually favors one direction, politely tell them to get their act together and try the other side too. The text will not necessarily say, "Swap over and let the other player do it" or "now do it the other way." Assume that this is what partner training means. Both players do all techniques in both directions with both legs. To avoid brain-numbing repetition, this won't be written in the exercise instruction text, so it is being written now.

Cavalete

Many of these routines can be done alone or with a partner. You will notice that if a player is alone, use of a cavalete is sometimes suggested. A cavalete is a wooden rack, approximately 1m 10cm (3 feet 8 inches) tall, and 50cm (1 foot, 8 inches) wide. It is not like a kung fu dummy in that you are not meant to strike it. Rather it's a focus to move around or kick over the top of.

This cavalete can be constructed easily out of wood. You don't have to wait to build a cavalete to begin training. Lack of a cavalete is never a good enough reason to avoid training a movement. The back of a chair will work almost as well, or even a pile of cushions or indeed nothing at all except the idea of a target. The point is to use something a little over waist height and around the same width as a human body to practice your moves around.

So choose what you like with these exercises. Some exercises have an **A** for advanced or an **I** for intermediate next to them. This means that these exercises or games include movements from those sections of this book; or maybe the way they are combined is better suited for players with some experience. Exercises with no **A** or **I** are suitable for everybody. These letters give a general idea about who the exercises might interest. Having said this, such categories are only loose guidelines. People are usually able to decide for themselves whether a sequence is for them yet or not. Some beginners get the hang of movements in the **A** section surprisingly quickly. This author's six-year-old daughter can do some movements in the **A** section which he steers clear of.

The movements in each exercise sequence are identified according to their corresponding number in the Movement section (Part 1). So in an exercise involving ginga, the ginga is identified by a (No. 1) in parentheses, or an exercise including meia lua de frente will show (No. 21), etc. Readers can turn to the movement description and study it. If you are not sure what is going on in any description, it's useful to take some time to study the appropriate photos and calculate for yourself how the moves will fit together. This is educational and adds to an appreciation of strategy.

East-West

Sometimes, to explain directions, the text will say "East" and "West." This is not really East and West, so you won't need a compass. East/West merely symbolize opposite directions. This is to avoid over-complex written instructions bogged down by the words left and right (which denote not only directions but also limbs). East and West is often much simpler, believe me. If it says in an exercise that the kick goes west and the negativa lateral goes west, this means that the head of the negativa goes west. Why? If your head went east it would run bang into the west-moving kick.

The Comfort Zone

Challenge yourself and step out of your comfort zone once in a while. Some students like to play upright and do high kicks and acrobatics. These players can benefit from playing low. Those who like to play low can reverse that by practicing a few parafusos, armada puladas, and upright kicks. If you never do macacos, resolve to include one or two in each game until they become second nature. This keeps us growing and adds new dimensions to the capoeira jogo. The same applies to tempo. If we play slowly all the time, then slow is the only speed we end up being able to play. So play fast, play slow, play up, play down, play in and play out to become the most versatile capoeirista you can be.

A Final Thought

Train for yourself. The only person we really overcome in the roda is oneself anyway. This is not the same as being selfish. There's a very big place for generosity. Yet to paraphrase some wise advice, "we are not here to live up to other people's expectations, nor are they here to live up to ours."

If you see great capoeira players and become totally inspired, that's fantastic. Yet never get dispirited by seeing great capoeira or being around people much better than you. Capoeira, like many skills, is learned most effectively by just showing up. Sometimes rodas don't seem very democratic, though capoeira is for everybody, from the know-nothing new beginner to the Mestre of Mestres. The bottom line with this training is to have fun.

It's idleness, it's vadiação, so let's go, let's play capoeira!

Sequences to Do Alone or with a Partner

Please note that the numbers in parentheses under each exercise in Part 2 correspond to the numbers of the specific basic movements involved *as listed and described in Part 1 of this book*. Where alternative movements are possible—as, for example, with different types of aú quebrado or different types of bananeira—the corresponding numbers are depicted with a slash between them. To illustrate, in the Movement section (Part 1), aú normal is No. 16, and two types of cabeçada are Nos. 84 and 87. Thus an exercise sequence in Part 2 involving cabeçada against aú normal would provide reference numbers for more details on the specific moves in the following way: (Nos.16, 84/87). You therefore know that you have a choice of two cabeçadas that you can practice.

1. Rabo de Arraia—Negativa Lateral under kick

■ (TWO PLAYERS) (NOS. 33, 8)

Player 1 kicks rabo de arraia west, and Player 2 ducks down low under the kicking foot, in a negativa lateral (head directed west, away from the kick). Do this randomly too, so Player 2 doesn't know which direction the kick will come from.

Pointers

Both players can ginga before the rabo de arraia is delivered. Kick slightly to the fore of your partner, so the kicking foot passes directly over their body as they negativa lateral. Remember when you do any esquiva (escape technique), negativa lateral included, the head is moving away from the kicking foot, not toward it.

✺

2. Meia Lua de Compasso

■ (TWO PLAYERS) (NO. 32)

Player 1 does meia lua de compasso and is followed very closely by Player 2 doing the same movement. They kick over each other's body, return to an upright position, and repeat 5 times, then change direction.

Pointers

Both players will be moving in the same direction, so if Player 1 kicks with the left foot, Player 2 will kick with the right. Player 1 stays down until after Player 2's kick has passed over. The kicking legs will form a cross over their bodies at the top of the kick. Vary the speed and try to go as rapidly as possible while still in control. You can do this alone over a cavalete for practice.

✺

3. (I) Aú Normal—Cabeçada

■ (TWO PLAYERS) (NOS. 16, 84/87)

Player 1 does the aú and Player 2 answers by aiming a cabeçada at Player 1's belly while they are upside down.

Pointers

Just touch your head to the belly and don't smash the oppoent over. Work on your timing so that you hit the target when they are fully upside down.

⁂

4. Bênção—Chapa de Costas

■ (NOS. 20, 26/27)

Do a bênção, bring the leg back, and immediately kick again with chapa de costas, using the same leg.

Pointers

Try to follow the bênção as closely as possible with the chapa de costas. Do this against a partner or a cavalete. Once you feel confident with the sequence, as the leg comes back out of bênção, convert it into a chapa de costas without letting the foot return to the ground between the two kicks.

⁂

5. (I) Bênção into Chapa de Costas— up into Bananeira

■ (NOS. 20, 26/27, 41/42/43)

Do a bênção, bring the leg back, and immediately kick again with chapa de costas, using the same leg. Without returning the kicking foot to the floor, push up into bananeira.

Pointers

After the chapa de costas, make a smooth push into bananeira and try to hold the position for a while, or walk forward and backward on your hands.

⁂

6. (I) Queixada 2—Armada—Meia Lua de Compasso to the left and right

■ (NOS. 18, 19, 32, 100)

This can be done with a partner or alone with a cavalete. With a partner, Player 1 starts with queixada, Player 2 follows with queixada, and so on thoughout the movements. If you use a cavalete, kick over it, joining the three kicks seamlessly, one following the other.

Pointers

Do the movements close to your partner and use your esquiva and bent waist to avoid being kicked. Vary the speed, but keep the sequence smooth and under control. It is not necessary to ginga to change direction, as your front foot has automatically changed due to the sequence.

☀

7. (I) Queixada—Armada—Meia Lua de Compasso—Aú Normal/Compasso

■ (NOS. 18, 19, 32, 15/16)

This is the same sequence, though Player 1 continues **in the same direction** as their final meia lua de compasso with an aú, while Player 2 does aú **in the opposite direction** to their final meia lua de compasso kick. In this way, while the two players' kicks have all been rotating in unison like two vertical cogs turning together, the aús follow one after the other around the perimeter of an imaginary circle on the floor to avoid crashing together.

Pointers

After the meia lua, your foot is at the back. Take it to a parallel again to help you launch for the aú. Study the relevant movements in the first section of this book to get a feel for the techniques you'll be doing. Passada, or footwork, is not a precise science or an immovable statue. Configure your feet between techniques in a way that is best for you to achieve your objective.

✸

8. Armada—Esquiva together

■ (TWO PLAYERS) (NO. 19; SEE FIG. 8 IN NO. 100 FOR AN EXAMPLE OF THE APPROPRIATE ESQUIVA)

Two players do armadas in unison. Player 1 turns armada with the right foot kicking. Player 2 esquivas by bending the back left leg, then turns an armada, kicking with the left leg (and Player 1 esquivas). Go around and around for 5 alternating kicks each.

Pointers

You should be within kicking range of the partner the whole time. It is the esquiva that enables you to turn fast precise kicks in close proximity without crashing into each other.

✸

9. Queixadas Alternating with a Partner

■ (NO. 18) OR (NO. 100, FIGS. 1–4)

With a partner, or over a cavalete, do front-leg queixadas from side to side. If you are with a partner, begin standing on your imaginary line. Player 1 steps forward and kicks with their queixada, Player 2 esquivas. Player 2 queixadas, Player 1 esquivas. Continue until tired, then ginga to get your breath back and repeat.

Pointers

Get into a groove and try to build speed and precision while remaining close to the other player. This is a great stamina builder, so persist until you are tired before quitting. You do not need to ginga, as the queixada changes direction for you.

❂

10. Negativa Normal—Tesoura

■ (NOS. 5, 95)

Drop into a negativa normal—let's say with the left leg extended and weight on the left support hand. Throw the right leg and hand over and lower yourself into a low tesoura, horizontal to the ground. Push back with the tesoura.

Pointers

Remember the phrase, *Calça engomada, não toca no chão.* Play very low, iron the trousers, don't touch the floor.

❂

11. Player 1: Negativa Normal—Tesoura Player 2: Aú Normal/Compasso

■ (NOS. 5, 95/96, 15/16)

Player 1 will do the same as in the previous exercise, toward Player 2. As Player 1 closes in, Player 2 does aú clean away from the tesoura, drops into negativa, and slides tesoura in toward Player 1, who answers with aú and does the same thing on other side.

Pointers

Both players keep moving all the time. Don't collapse on your stomach in tesoura, but make a point of completing the movement. After your partner has escaped with their aú, push up from the tesoura position into a cocorinha (without putting your knees on the ground), and stand up.

❖

12. (I) Armada—Rasteira

■ (TWO PLAYERS) (NOS. 19, 54)

Player 1 does armada. Player 2 rasteiras beneath it, with the head moving away from the kick. Do to the left and then right 10 times (5 times each direction) and change.

Pointers

Rasteira with your body low. As the kick swings around, you are turning your back to the kicking foot. If you are offering your chest and face to the kick, then you are doing the rasteira in the wrong direction. The rasteira is essentially an extension of an esquiva. The long, straightened leg sweeps in a clean arc along the ground, like a scythe. Stop at the very point you hit the back of the other player's foot. This should happen while their kick is still in the air, probably directly above your head. The rasteira is much more effective if the opponent has only one foot on the ground. It is even more effective if you sweep the supporting foot at the exact moment it is swiveling around during the armada kick. Don't take the opponent down, unless it's by pre-agreement and they are experienced enough to know how to fall into a negativa.

❖

13. (I) Martelo de Estalo—Rasteira

■ (TWO PLAYERS) (NOS. 30, 3, 54)

This is a similar routine to the last exercise, except here Player 1 kicks with martelo de estalo. Player 2 esquivas away and under the kick, drops very low, and sweeps behind the support foot.

Pointers

Coordinate bending low and sweeping so that they happen simultaneously.

✦

14. (I) Armada—Rasteira—Aú Normal

■ (TWO PLAYERS) (NOS. 19, 54, 16)

Player 1 does armada east, and Player 2 does rasteira east. As soon as Player 1 feels the sweeping foot hit the outside of their own foot, he or she leans (west) and does an aú normal over the sweeping leg.

Pointers

Take this slowly at first to get the feel of it, and be careful not to aú off balance and fall on top of the person who did the rasteira. Try to aú over rasteira straight from armada, **before** the kicking leg has touched back to the ground. Make the changeover transitions smooth, so Players 1 and 2 become like a machine of perpetual motion.

✦

15. (I) Armada—Parafuso

■ (TWO PLAYERS) (NOS. 19, 79/80)

Player 1 does armada east then Player 2 does armada east, Player 1 does another armada east, Player 2 does parafuso east.

Pointers

Play close together and esquiva from the armadas. Player 2 will have a better position for parafuso if he or she begins the turn for that kick with the kicking leg at the back, so the kick can launch after a 180° turn. Twist at the waist, pivot on the feet, and attempt to parafuso over Player 1. Be light and very relaxed in your limbs as you do parafuso. If you have no partner, kick over a cavalete.

✸

16. (I) Martelo de Estalo—Aú Coisa

■ (TWO PLAYERS) (NOS. 30, 45)

Player 1 aims a martelo de estalo at Player 2. Player 2 esquivas into an aú coisa aimed at the belly of Player 1.

Pointers

Player 2 will have to esquiva and aú with concentration, both to the side and inward. Aim to esquiva into optimal position to kick your aú coisa directly at Player 1. Work on setting your body distance and the angle of your legs correctly to direct the soles of both feet together against the other player's abdomen. Having kicked, don't fall forward, but pull the feet back and continue in the aú to come out to the side, one foot at a time.

✸

17. (A) Armada—Helicóptero

■ (TWO PLAYERS) (NOS. 19, 76)

Player 1 armadas west. In this exercise Player 2 responds to Player 1's armada with a helicóptero.

when doing any sequence of movements, no matter what they are or how many techniques are in the sequence.

❖

21. (I) Aú—Negativa Normal—Chapéu de Couro

■ (NOS. 16, 5, 48)

If you were to aú to the left, upon landing, extend your left leg into a negativa normal and immediately swing it up to continue into chapéu de couro to the left.

Pointers

If you aú left, the first foot to come off the ground is the right foot. Land on this right foot out of the aú, bend the right knee, and drop immediately into negativa normal with your left leg extended. Keep your support (left) hand close to your backside and throw the left leg up to swing the left then the right foot over a cavalete with chapéu de couro.

❖

22. (I) Player 1: Armada
Player 2: Esquiva Lateral—Aú—Negativa Normal—Change Direction—Chapéu de Couro

■ (NOS. 19, 3, 16, 5, 48)

Now is a good time to set the chapéu de couro into a sequence with a partner. Player 1 kicks with armada east. Player 2 esquiva laterals under it, straight into aú and negativa normal, all to the east. The switch comes here. Player 2 has his or her east-side leg extended in the negativa normal, and the east-side hand on the floor.

But Player 1 is to the west. Player 2 swaps hands for support on the ground, and swaps support foot and extended leg, so that he or she is now in negativa normal the other way. Kick chapéu de couro over Player 1.

Pointers

Practice a smooth changeover of hands and feet when you change direction in negativa normal. Remember, you can be on a flat support foot in negativa normal, or on the ball of your support foot, whichever you prefer. Do the chapéu de couro as soon as you have swapped the negativa. Player 1 can just ginga after armada and esquiva as necessary when the chapéu de couro comes his way.

✺

23. (A) Player 1: Armada
Player 2: Resistençia—Rolé
Player 1: Aú Chibata

■ (NOS. 19, 88, 13, 59)

Player 1 kicks with an armada east, Player 2 drops into resistençia and rolés east, followed closely by Player 1 leaping east into an aú chibata.

Pointers

After the armada, and just before throwing for the chibata, bring your feet together and jump from two feet, as described in the Movement section (see No. 59). To make this exercise more unpredictable, Player 2 can vary whether they rolé east or west after their resistençia, forcing Player 1 to think and act quickly as he launches the aú chibata.

✺

24. (I) Aú Batendo

■ (NO. 47)

Have a partner hold out one arm and extend the hand, palm up, just below shoulder level. Focus on the palm of his hand and do an aú batendo, bringing the top of your foot down lightly on the palm of the outstretched hand. As soon as you have kicked the hand, bring your kicking leg back and come out of the aú to the side.

Pointers

Work on controlling the movement in a momentary bananeira as you execute the kick. Do not let your kicking foot just flop forward and hit the hand on its way to the ground, but kick it lightly and with control, and then continue on your way out of the aú.

✳

25. Meia Lua de Compasso— Martelo Giratório

■ (TWO PLAYERS) (NOS. 32, 31)

Player 1 does the kick east; Player 2 follows straight after and in the same direction.

Pointers

Players can do this as a set sequence or just play ginga, with Player 1 kicking meia lua de compasso toward Player 2 when he or she feels like it, and Player 2 responding by ducking in and following Player 1's kicking leg with his own martelo giratório.

✳

26. (I) Player 1: Corta Capim—Meia Lua de Compasso—Vingativa
Player 2: Ginga—Esquiva Lateral

■ (NOS. 36, 2, 32, 3, 92)

Player 1 does two, three, or four spins of corta capim with the right leg. Player 2 does ginga.

At the end of the final corta capim, Player 1 brings his right foot to the ground directly in front of Player 2. Player 1 aims meia lua de compasso at Player 2 with the left leg. Player 2 does esquiva under the kick. (Player 2's right hand will be on the floor as he leans over to the right, with the left hand defending his face.) Player 1 brings his kicking (left) leg back to where it started. As Player 2 begins to rise up out of the esquiva lateral, Player 1 slips in with his right leg behind Player 2's legs and instantly levers the opponent over with vingativa.

Pointers

To best position himself for the vingativa, Player 1 should bring his meia lua kicking leg way back, almost in line with the two feet of Player 2. Study the picture of vingativa in the Movement section (see No. 92), and visualize what you would have to do to get into that position directly after a meia lua de compasso.

❄

27. Armada—Tesoura 1

■ (TWO PLAYERS) (NOS. 19, 93)

Player 1 does armada. Player 2 does a slight esquiva and jumps into a tesoura just as Player 1 returns his or her kicking leg to the back again.

Pointers

The best moment to do a tesoura is the exact point when the opponent completes a technique and is not fully balanced again. If they are doing ginga and you line yourself up for tesoura, they will probably see it coming. If they are just returning their kicking leg to the ground after armada and you leap in and entrap and lever, you probably have them.

Note: You may want to practice this on mats. Concentrate on finding the best angle and most direct route for your leap in.

❂

28. (I) Player 1: Rabo de Arraia
Player 2: Esquiva Queda de Rins—Rolé

■ (NO. 33, 38, 13/14)

Player 1 does a rabo de arraia; Player 2 drops beneath it into esquiva queda de rins, and comes out with rolé.

Pointers

In this esquiva queda de rins the elbow into your hip will be on the side facing (or closest to) your partner, so then you can still see them when you do the movement. If you did it with your arm on the other side, it would force you to turn away from them.

❂

29. Armada—Resistençia

■ (TWO PLAYERS) (NOS. 19, 88)

Player 1, armada east

Player 2, resistençia

Player 2, armada east

Player 1, resistência

Player 1, armada west

Player 2, resistência

Player 2, armada west

Player 1, resistência

Repeat the cycle until you are out of breath and beyond. Work your body and feel the twist of the waist with the armada.

Pointers

Get into a rhythm with this exercise and use it to build timing and stamina together. Make sure you go all the way down into resistência, and the player doing armada should kick low enough to ensure that the defender has to go all the way down. Be springy and light on your feet throughout the sequence.

❂

30. (A) Player 1: Armada
Player 2: Cocorinha—Armada Pulada

■ (NOS. 19, 10, 78)

Player 1 armadas east. Player 2 drops into cocorinha, back halfway against the kick, so facing northeast. As soon as the armada passes over, Player 2 springs straight up into a jumping armada pulada (east), aimed at the head of Player 1.

Pointers

When you do armada pulada, remember to bring the second leg (the non-kicking leg) high as you turn in the kick. When you land in this exercise, you can land standing or back into cocorinha and then up into ginga.

❂

31. (I) Player 1: Meia Lua de Frente
Player 2: Esquiva Lateral—Resistençia—Macaco

■ (NOS. 21, 3, 70)

Player 1 does meia lua de frente west. Player 2 does esquiva lateral west, then swings the extended leg west and drops into resistençia (with the hand nearest to Player 1 on the floor) and macacos east.

Pointers

Swinging the extended leg from an esquiva and jumping back into macaco is an excellent method of changing direction in capoeira. Look at your partner while you macaco, which will mean you must have the resistençia hand on the floor on their side. (See figs. 1 and 2 in No. 70, Movement section.) If you put your far hand on the floor first you will be looking away from the opponent.

❋

32. Player 1: Martelo de Estalo
Player 2: Esquiva—Chapa

■ (NOS. 30, 4, 24)

Player 1 does a martelo de estalo. Player 2 esquivas inward and forward. Once in a good position from esquiva, Player 2 aims a chapa directly at the center of Player 1's chest.

Pointers

If Player 1 does the martelo de estalo kicking with the right foot, it would be coming at Player 2's left side. Therefore Player 2 will esquiva right, and kick chapa with the left foot. Player 2: Look at the target before you kick, and sink your weight down into your support foot when you do the chapa.

Note: Player 2 may have to jump sideways into the esquiva to get a good clean central position and open shot at Player 1's chest. Find these openings by doing esquiva with enough reach (or leap) to create them yourself.

※

33. Player 1: Martelo de Estalo
Player 2: Esquiva—Cabeçada

■ (NOS. 30, 4, 84)

Player 1 does a martelo de estalo. Player 2 esquivas inward and forward. Once in a good position from the esquiva, Player 2 aims a cabeçada directly at the center of Player 1's chest.

Pointers

This begins in the same way as the previous sequence, though it requires two steps to achieve cabeçada. If Player 1 does the martelo de estalo with the right leg, Player 2 does one step/esquiva to the right. Player 2 will be leaning over his bent right leg, and should try to get that bent right leg well lined up in front of the kicking player. The chest is your target, so work on positioning yourself front and center in a single bound with the esquiva.

The second step, toward Player 1 with the left foot, will enable Player 2 to strike at the chest with a high cabeçada. To recap, Player 1 does the martelo, and Player 2 leaps with esquiva then steps in toward Player 1 to deliver a cabeçada with the top of the head. When doing this cabeçada you can cross your arms under your face to defend against joelhada or other kicks.

※

34. (I) Negativa Lateral—Moenda— Aú Cabeça no Chão

■ (NOS. 8, 44, 34)

This can be done by one player, or two mirroring each other. Do negativa lateral west, then moenda west, and without lifting the head from the floor, aú cabeça no chão east.

Pointers

Breathe naturally but deeply during this sequence. The aim here is to link all three of these movements so that they segue, one to the other, in a very smooth and efficient way. You should be looking forward at your partner, or if you are alone, at a cavalete, 100% of the time throughout the sequence.

❂

35. Reverse Armadas

■ (TWO PLAYERS) (NO. 19)

Two players stand close and within kicking distance of each other. Both do armadas. The exercise here is to rotate the armadas in opposite directions while coordinating them. Player 1 does armada west, and then Player 2 does armada east. The esquivas are the same, just tilting back far enough to avoid the kick. Do five kicks, alternating between Player 1 and 2 (so ten in all) and then both players change direction and do the sequence the other way.

Pointers

This exercise forces you to concentrate on timing. If you are out of time, your legs will crash in the middle, so Player 2 has to make sure that he does not kick until Player 1's armada has passed by and vice versa.

❂

36. Reverse Meia Lua de Compasso

■ (TWO PLAYERS) (NO. 32)

This is exactly the same exercise as the last one, except this is more difficult because the players are doing meia lua de compasso, a movement that leaves an even narrower opportunity to reverse the kick against the other player. Alternate 10 kicks, Player 1 west, Player 2 east.

Pointers

Play close, and keep the meia lua kicking leg totally straight when you kick. Bending the kicking leg to make this exercise work is not an option. The purpose is to fine-tune your timing, and if you do sloppy meia lua de compassos with bent kicking legs you are selling yourself short on the training. Remember also that your head should always be back throughout the meia lua de compasso. Do not let it swing to the front as you return to a standing position. The head must come up, yes, but not so far forward that it is an open target for a kick.

✦

37. Martelo de Estalo Drill

■ (TWO PLAYERS) (NO. 30)

Here's a drill to loosen your hips up and strengthen your martelos. Stand facing a partner, about a meter apart. Both players stand with legs splayed in good balance, a little wider than shoulder width apart.

Player 1 does a martelo de estalo kick to the other player's right shoulder with the left foot, then returns the foot to its original position. Immediately Player 2 martelo kicks Player 1's right shoulder with the left foot and returns it to the ground. Immediately Player 1 martelos Player 2's left shoulder with the right foot, returning it to its base; and Player 2 answers by doing martelo to Player 1's left shoulder with the right foot.

The players are alternating direction each time and getting into a rhythm.

Pointers

The martelo is a powerful kick. Your partner's shoulder is a focus area and not a heavy bag. If you want to build power in your kicks by repeatedly kicking a target, your training partner's body is definitely not the target to choose.

Note: Remember that to kick martelo, it's necessary to swivel on your support foot to direct the toes of the support foot away from your partner. This will enable you to angle yourself to kick higher and more easily, without restriction in your pelvis. If the toes of your support foot are facing your partner, it will be impossible to get your knee high on the kicking leg.

✸

38. Martelo de Estalo—Aú Normal

■ (NOS. 30, 16)

This is an exercise for one player. Do a martelo de estalo west and before returning your kicking foot to the floor, drop the west-side hand to the floor and aú normal to the west. Repeat everything to the east.

Pointers

When you have done the martelo, keep the knee of your kicking leg in front of you, with the kick foot still up and the kicking leg bent, then focus on controlling your weight well as you bend the support leg until your hand touches the floor. Be solid and secure as you do this, then turn over immediately in the aú.

❋

39. (A) Esquiva Lateral— Negativa Normal—S-Dobrado

■ (NOS. 3, 5, 71/72)

Two players can coordinate this, or you can do it alone. Do esquiva lateral, and then swing the extended leg around in front of you for the negativa normal and S-dobrado.

Pointers

You're aiming for total fluidity of movement with this. Look to the front or toward a cavalete or a partner throughout the sequence to orient your position. From the esquiva lateral, if for example you had your right hand on the ground, you would shift over to left hand on the ground for negativa normal, and then throw the left leg up for the S-dobrado. Make all the transitions as seamless as you can.

❋

40. Player 1: Meia Lua de Frente— Aú Compasso
Player 2: Negativa Lateral— Queda de Rins—Tesoura

■ (NOS. 21, 15, 8, 37, 95)

Player 1 does meia lua de frente, slowly and low to the east. Player 2 does negativa lateral to the east. From that position, Player 2 draws their legs up in front of their body, supporting their body weight by tucking their elbow into their waist. (Please note that there is no specific photo of this position. It is a forward-facing queda de rins.) Player 2 then pushes forward with tesoura. Player 1 escapes with aú compasso.

Pointers

If Player 1 had kicked east with the right foot, Player 2 would do negativa lateral east and support their weight on their right elbow.

Player 2 does a different type of queda de rins. If you study the negativa lateral (No. 8), imagine the player staying this low but bending both legs sharply at the knee and tucking his waist directly onto his lower elbow. The soles of his two feet would face the front and be off the ground. (This technique can be seen on page 106 of the companion volume, *Capoeira Conditioning*). From that position, Player 2 launches the tesoura toward Player 1.

✺

41. Queixada—Meia Lua de Compasso: No-foot-down continuation sequence

■ (NOS. 18, 32)

Do a queixada and follow it with meia lua de compasso **without** returning the kicking leg to the ground between the two kicks.

Pointers

This works best when done fast. To make this even more challenging, do it with a partner, wherein both are coordinating the queixada—meia lua de compasso together.

✺

42. (I) Armada—Encruzilhada

■ (TWO PLAYERS) (NOS. 19, 53)

Player 1 does an armada west. Player 2 drops and spins with an encruzilhada (west), hooking the outside of Player 1's support foot when the kick is still in the air and approximately at its apex.

Pointers

If Player 1 does the armada with the right leg kicking, Player 2 will sweep/hook the outside of the opponent's support foot with the left leg. As soon as Player 2 senses Player 1 begin their kick, Player 2 must drop and spin instantly so that the back leg sweeps around to catch the opponent before they have completed their kick.

As usual with powerful sweeps in training, you can just show this by pulling it fractionally short of making contact with the other player's heel.

❀

43. Bênção—Negativa de Solo

■ (TWO PLAYERS) (NOS. 20, 6)

Player 1 kicks toward Player 2 with a bênção. Player 2 drops rapidly and hooks his extended leg behind the heel of Player 1's support foot.

Pointers

To sweep here, Player 2 gives the leg he has extended a short, sharp tug, hooked around Player 1's support foot, while Player 1 is still on one leg. To do this properly, both to avoid being kicked with the bênção and to get deep enough in to hook the negativa de solo, Player 2 will have to drop very quickly. The head goes backward and downward simultaneously, and the body weight is caught on the hands on the same side as the extended (hooking) leg.

❖

44. Negativa Lateral—Negativa de Solo 2: Lateral Swap-Over

■ (NOS. 8, 7)

Negativa lateral with head to the west. Push up with your hands and without standing up, cross the leg over in front of your body, so that you are in a negativa de solo 2, laterally with your head directed east.

Pointers

This is a good exercise for changing the direction of your esquivas rapidly and efficiently while remaining low to the ground. Even though there is a lot of muscular contraction involved in manipulating your body weight on your arms like this, remain fully relaxed and breathe deeply as you do it.

❖

45. (I) Negativa Lateral—Negativa de Solo 2: Lateral Swap-Over with Aú Cabeça no Chão

■ (NOS. 8, 7, 34)

This begins the same as the previous exercise. This time you will add aú cabeça no chão after the negativa de solo 2, so that you can link everything together without coming into an upright position.

This is the order: negativa lateral west, change and negativa de solo with head pointing east. Continue in an aú cabeça no chão east, then straight into negativa lateral east, swap negativa de solo with head west, segueing into aú cabeça no chão west.

The full cycle has six movements in total.

Pointers

This can be done alone, and it is also fun to try it with a partner, mirroring each other's movements. The transition from negativa de solo into aú cabeça no chão can be a bit tricky for some people. Concentrate on creating a good base with your head and two hands. The main thing is to be small from the negativa de solo. Bend your legs, bend your arms, and get all the potentially unwieldy body parts and limbs in close to your center so you have more control over them. Keep your slightly bent legs in front of you and roll over on your head so you fall into negativa lateral in the other direction.

＊

46. (I) Rabo de Arraia—Negativa Lateral and Negativa de Solo 2: Lateral Swap-Over with Aú Cabeça no Chão

■ (TWO PLAYERS) (NOS. 33, 8, 7, 34)

This is done with a partner. Player 1 aims the kicking foot of a rabo de arraia at Player 2's head. Player 2 escapes from the foot in negativa lateral. So Player 1 swaps legs and aims another rabo de arraia in the other direction, also at Player 2's head. Player 2 swaps into negativa de solo as described in the previous two sequences, and continues over with aú cabeça no chão.

Pointers

Player 1: Aim your kicks directly at the target. Even if you are only showing the kicks, it is always good form to aim them directly. If you don't direct kicks, it is never really necessary to esquiva, as they are going to pass over the opponent anyway. If the kick doesn't relate to the target, and the esquiva doesn't relate to the kick, it means that people are just throwing their legs about randomly, which makes things less interesting.

✷

47. Player 1: Meia Lua de Compasso Player 2: Cocorinha—Cabeçada

■ (NOS. 32, 10, 84)

Player 1 does a meia lua de compasso, and Player 2 ducks under it with a low cocorinha. As soon as the kick has passed over Player 2's head he or she aims a cabeçada at Player 1's open chest or abdomen.

Pointers

Any time a player does a kick in capoeira, there is a chance that they leave themselves exposed in some way or other. The meia lua de compasso or rabo de arraia often presents such a moment of vulnerability, just after the kick has passed. On the other hand, as the kick may be done at high speed, this opening won't necessarily be there for long. Practice this sequence to be aware of the opening, to deliberately look for it, and to rapidly exploit it with a cabeçada.

✷

48. Looking for an Opening under Meia Lua de Compasso

■ (TWO PLAYERS) (NO. 100, FIG. 9)

Two players do meia lua de compasso.

In No. 100 (in the Movement section, Part 1), both players are doing a sequence of coordinated meia lua de compasso movements. We can borrow fig. 9 from that sequence of photos to show that if the player on the right didn't aim his kick over his partner (as in fig. 10), but instead aimed it under her, it would have found her body quite open.

Player 1: Kick a meia lua de compasso. Player 2: Follow 'round with a rabo de arraia, timed and aimed to attack the open area of Player 1's body. To defend against this, Player 2 will either have to immediately stamp his own kicking leg down to the ground in front and turn to create a wall against the incoming kick, or, if Player 2 is quick, she could roll away from the kick into a queda de quatro—rolé.

✵

49. High-Repetition Rasteira

■ (NO. 54)

With a partner or alone using a cavalete, practice doing ginga and dropping into rasteira then coming back up to ginga. If you have taken the right foot back in ginga, when it comes back to center, sweep rasteira with the left foot. Immediately bring the left foot to the center, do two ginga, and as you bring the left foot from the back to the center, drop for a rasteira with the right foot.

Pointers

Do high repetitions of these rasteiras—between 50 and 100 (or more)—to build stamina, strength in your legs, speed, and excellent timing when doing the sweep. Vary the height of your torso as you sweep the foot, making it sometimes medium, sometimes very low. You can also vary whether you put a support hand on the ground or do the rasteira with no hands on the ground.

✵

50. High-Repetition Armada taking the feet from a parallel stance

■ (NO. 19)

Stand with your feet about shoulder width apart and turn armada by robustly building momentum with a swing of the arms, shoulders, and waist. Armada side to side non-stop with good speed, and then rest by doing ginga. Repeat.

Pointers

This differs from the regular armada in that your foot begins the turn from the side of your body, not the back. Land your kicking foot back to the side again, shoulder width apart from the other one.

This requires a forceful twist of the waist and shoulders and good use of the arms for momentum sufficient to catapult the leg around. Make sure that you kick with a straight leg and get into a good rhythm. Rocking from side to side by shifting the weight from foot to foot increases the speed of the kicks too. This is a great workout for your oblique muscles and will burn fat around your waist, as well as building stamina and increasing speed in your armada kicks. You can kick over a cavalete, or better still, do this together with a partner, coordinating your movements by doing side esquivas with no hands on the floor (No. 4) when the other player's kick is passing over.

✳

51. (I) Aú Cruzado—Negativa Normal—Chapéu de Couro

■ (NOS. 35, 5, 48)

This is a good one to do with a cavalete. Aú cruzado off your left foot, so your left leg crosses over in front of your body and you land again on your left foot. Your right leg will still be in the air at this point (see fig. 4, No. 35).

Now, instead of coming up into ginga, pass the right leg through the gap between your hands and the left foot (see fig. 4, No. 35) and fall into negativa normal with your right hand on the floor. Immediately swing the right leg up and over the cavalete in a chapéu de couro to the right.

Pointers

If you do this with a partner, pass the aú cruzado over their body when they are in a negativa lateral, rolé, or some such maneuver, and then pass the leg through as described above, fall into negativa normal, and swing the chapéu de couro at your partner as they rise up into ginga. Keep your support hand close to your backside in the negativa normal, and center your weight over it to give you a stable support for the swing into chapéu de couro.

✦

52. Chapa no Chão—Esquiva para Trás

■ (TWO PLAYERS) (NOS. 28, 4)

This is an exercise for timing, speed, and stamina. Both players stand facing the same way. Player 1 does chapa no chão east. Player 2 does esquiva back away from the chapa (east). Player 2 steps forward and does chapa no chão west; Player 1 does esquiva to the back (west).

Both players turn around and face the other way, then continue the cycle as before. After one kick, one escape each, they turn again, and repeat. Do this until out of breath to build stamina.

Pointers

Aim the chapa no chão robustly at your partner, forcing them to literally jump back into the esquiva. Build into a good rhythm so you move back and forth, turn, back and forth, turn, etc.

Even though the esquiva No. 4 can be used for turning kicks, it can also be used to esquiva back away from a front kick, with the small adaptation of stepping and leaning backward rather than sideways.

Note: Step forward for the chapa no chão and put your hand on the floor at the very moment that the leg snaps out into the kick.

❖

53. (A) Rabo de Arraia—Mola

■ (TWO PLAYERS) (NOS. 32/33, 73)

Player 1 aims a rabo de arraia or meia lua de compasso at Player 2. Player 2 leaps back as the kick passes over him and lands on the shoulders, then springs back to the feet with mola.

Pointers

This is a good sequence for demonstrations, especially if Players 1 and 2 coordinate the meia luas and molas and repeat the movement two or three times.

❖

Focus Games

54. Jogo de Baixo (Low Game)

■ (NOS. 1, 2, 5, 6, 7, 9, 10, 11, 13, 14, AND 15; 34 AND 37 ARE
OPTIONAL INTERMEDIATE TECHNIQUES)

Playing on the ground

Play a capoeira game, using ginga, the various negativa movements,
cocorinha, resistência, rolé, queda de quatro, queda de rins, aú cabeça
no chão, tesoura, and aú compasso.

Pointers

No kicks! Just the movements specified above. Practice moving around
on the ground. Play this alone with a cavalete or with a partner. Only
touch the ground with your hands and feet (or head for intermediate
players). Use the rolé and aú cabeça no chão to circle and change
direction. Keep moving all the time and don't stay in one spot.

❂

55. Jogo de Dentro

Make a restricted-size circle, no bigger than 2 meters (6.5 feet) in
diameter, and play capoeira inside it with a partner.

Pointers

Move steadily all the time and don't crash or become entangled with
the other player. Watch your head, keeping it protected by your body
position and hands while doing ginga. The two players shouldn't be
knocking foreheads as they ginga, even in a restricted space. Attempt
to find openings of exposed face, belly, chest, and ribs and aim kicks

at them. Achieving a clean attack on an open target, particularly attacks that are unanticipated and completely surprise your opponent, is a strategic goal. Remember the lyric, *Devagar, devagarinho, cuidado com o seu pezinho* (Take it slowly and calmly, be careful with your foot).

❂

56. (I) Floreios and Acrobacia (Flourishes and Acrobatics)

◾ (NOS. 16, 48, 36, 46, 59, 61, 62, 63, 64, 65, 66, 67, 68, 70, 71, 72, 73, 74, 75, 76, 77, 78, 79, 80, 81)

With a partner, in a regular-size roda, no bigger than 6 meters (20 feet) in diameter, play a game of ginga and do all the acrobatics or floreios that you know. Have no self-consciousness and don't worry if they don't work. The point of training is to train; if you got it right the first time then you wouldn't need to practice. If you can only do aú, then go for that.

Pointers

Try some jumping kicks like armada pulada and parafuso, as well as aú quebrado and pião de mão. It's time to give macaco and chapéu de couro a spin around the block too. You have more space in this roda, but stay in sync with your partner, and link floreios in a game that stays within striking range of your opponent. Play in rhythm to whatever music you play.

❂

57. Playing in Slow Motion

There is an exercise doing aú normal in slow motion. This takes it a step further to play a whole game in slow motion. Not just a bit slower than usual, but as slow as you can go and still remain moving.

Pointers

As you see a technique coming toward you, there is now plenty of time to think about it. Use this slow-motion opportunity to ask yourself why you are going to esquiva in a certain way, what counterattack you will use, where you will aim it and why? That's a lot of questions to ask in the course of a kick, but they say a game of capoeira is like a game of chess, so here is a chance to find out.

✦

58. Speed Play

Regardless of exercises, the best training for capoeira is capoeira. Put on some fast music, and play faster than you feel comfortable with. Don't play so fast that you are out of control, but be prepared to really sweat and push yourself beyond your normal tempo. If you are already fast, then play fast longer to build stamina.

Pointers

Begin normally to warm up, and then by pre-arrangement with a partner, or alone with a cavalete, play so fast that you are really gasping for breath. At this point slow down and play calmly to get your breath back, but keep playing. When you feel better, repeat the speed burst.

Note: The same principle that applies in running is true of capoeira—some people are naturally fast. When they train for speed they get even faster. Others are not so naturally fast, and when they train for speed, they also get faster. So do some speed training if you want to be faster.

✦

59. Game with One or Two Hands on the Floor

This exercise consists of a focus game where both players should have either one or two hands on the floor 100% of the time throughout the game.

Pointers

Always have one hand on the floor, even to do ginga.

✸

60. Cabeçada Drill

■ (NO. 87)

Two play a low game without kicks. This is similar to the first exercise in this section, except here one of the players is looking carefully for openings through which to aim a cabeçada (No. 87).

Pointers

Targets for the cabeçada in this exercise are the abdomen, the chest, and the ribs. If Player 2 is going to do the cabeçada, Player 1 should move about and attempt to remain closed up, without leaving these areas exposed. Never play so defensively that it inhibits the smooth flow of your movements.

✸

61. Aú Chase

■ (NOS. 15/16)

Inside a pre-arranged circle, Player 1 stands at the east point and Player 2 at the west. Moving around the outside of the circle, Player

1 attempts to catch up with Player 2 as Player 2 runs away. But neither player is running; they are only doing aús repeatedly. Player 1 can change direction and go the other way around the circle at any time, to which, of course, Player 2 will have to respond by changing direction as well.

Pointers

This works well for players of similar abilities and will really get your heart and lungs doing overtime. If one player is much faster than the other, increase the size of the circle, so they have to do more work to catch up with the slower player. Don't crash into your partner when you do catch up.

⁜

Conditioning and Strength Exercises

62. Tesoura Push-Ups

■ (NOS. 95, 9/10, 5)

Use your arms to push (or rather spring) up from tesoura into cocorinha or negativa normal; then drop into tesoura and bounce straight up again into cocorinha or negativa normal on the other side; then swing over into tesoura and hop up again.

Pointers

Only hands and feet touch the ground. To make this even more tiring, and to build even better stamina and strength, push along the ground for a meter or so in tesoura, then spring into cocorinha, and repeat.

✳

63. Tesoura Spring Push-Ups

■ (NOS. 95, 87, 9/10)

This one will get you into shape fast. You don't have to do it for long to get results. Get into cocorinha, and lunge forward for a cabeçada angola. Lower further, with your elbows close in to your sides, for the bottom position of a regular push-up. In this position, bounce yourself forward a few meters, then widen your legs a bit and push back in tesoura to your starting point. Spring up into cocorinha and repeat, this time looking over the other shoulder in tesoura.

Pointers

When you bounce forward, be on the toes of both feet, and keep the arms bent low at the elbow. Do not touch the ground with anything but your hands and feet. Stay low to the ground all the way through the sequence. For push-ups, you bounce forward with arms continually bent at the elbows. Each spring should propel you forward a short distance.

❁

64. Cocorinha Walk

■ (NO. 10)

To add to the workload of the previous exercise, after springing up from the tesoura at the end of the cycle, walk forward in cocorinha position, then walk back. Swivel on your feet and walk forward in the other direction, and walk back. Repeat until your thighs start to burn, then dive forward for another set of tesoura spring push-ups.

Pointers

In the cocorinha walk, it is as if you are walking up and down the lines of a large V painted on the floor. Up and down one line, swivel at the junction of the two lines, then up and down the other line. Squat low throughout the walk and keep your hands on either side of your head.

❁

65. Queda de Quatro Walk

■ (NO. 11)

A good exercise to combine with the cocorinha walk is a queda de quatro walk. Do two strolls in cocorinha up and down the lines of your imaginary V painted on the ground. When you get to the point of the V, drop back into queda de quatro and walk up and down the lines of the V in queda de quatro position. Forward then back, and forward then back up the other line. After completing that, shoot up and do the cocorinha again. Repeat the whole cycle as long as you can handle it.

Pointers

Keep your hands and feet quite close together in the queda de quatro walk. If you let your body unfold too much it will become sloppy and slow.

✺

66. (A) Aú Normal in Slow Motion

■ (NO. 16)

This is what it says: a regular aú normal done at the slowest speed you can do it. Picture yourself as if you have been filmed doing this in slow motion.

Pointers

Warm up by doing some regular cartwheels and then get successively slower with each aú you do. Try to stop at the top of the position in a bananeira (No. 41) and then slowly lower the toes of your leading leg to the ground while holding the bananeira.

✺

67. Negativa de Solo 2: Lateral Jumping Push-Ups

■ (NO. 7)

This is a strength, springiness, and stamina builder *par excellence*. Drop into negativa de solo with the extended leg and foot pointing east. Push up onto your feet powerfully, jumping both feet off the ground. As you land, drop directly into negativa de solo with the extended leg and foot pointing west. Repeat, east to west to east, etc., until too tired to continue.

Pointers

To get a feel for this exercise, begin slowly without the jump. Work on sliding the leg and lowering your body into the negativa de solo with good control on your arms. Don't cheat yourself by not going all the way down and completing the movement. As soon as you are in position, push off with your arms, slide up again, and repeat to the other side, paying similar attention to form. When you are confident, push up hard enough that you jump high and powerfully off the ground between each negativa de solo.

✵

68. Aú Push-Up—Aú Queda de Rins Push-Up

A less advanced way to build strength in your arms, back, chest, and shoulders is to simply side-esquiva and lift one leg as if you are about to do an aú normal, then lower the top of your head to the ground and push up again until your arms are straight. Do this 10 or 20 times to the left, and the same to the right.

Pointers

You can experiment to make this an excellent waist stretcher by aligning both your hands on the ground with your body, and when you come to the full up position, stretch your raised leg back and squeeze your buttock, exhale, and flex your abs and squeeze your oblique muscle before inhaling and going down into the next rep.

To add variation, when you go to the down position, bend your neck so your lower ear brushes the floor while you rest your waist on your inner elbow in queda de rins and immediately push up to the top position. Your upper leg remains high the whole time. Do 10 reps on each side.

※

69. (I) Cabeça no Chão Waist Flexor
■ (NO. 40)

Hold a cabeça no chão. Point the toes of both feet, legs very straight, splayed out either side to the front of your body (only the head and hands touch the floor). In small movements, touch the big toe of the right foot to the floor, then bend and touch the big toe of the left foot to the floor. Alternate, bending and flexing your waist, while remaining standing on your head only (supported by your hands of course).

Pointers

Don't take your toes to the floor to help support your weight. This is only to train control of your movements while in the cabeça no chão position. Repeat the alternating waist bend 10 or 20 times. Do some loose gingas to relax your neck upon completion.

※

70. Cabeça no Chão Twister (with Moenda)
■ (NOS. 40, 8, 44)

Cabeça no chão, and splay your legs with the toes pointed. Twisting your waist, take your right leg across the front of your body and touch the left wrist with your toes, then twist the other way and touch your right wrist with the toes of your left foot. The only thing that touches the ground is your hands and head. Do 10 reps, drop to one side into negativa lateral and turn a moenda one way, then turn it back the other way.

Pointers

This is a full multi gym in a sequence and you don't have to leave the spot you are in. Do this when your body is already warm.

✴

71. Negativa (no hands)

■ (NOS. 2, 5)

Start with one leg forward, one back, as in No. 2, fig. 1, for example. From here, drop back into negativa normal (No. 5), but do not put either of your hands on the floor. If we take fig. 1 (No. 2) as our example, the player would bend his left leg deeper, squatting on his left leg, with his right leg extended to the front, as in No. 5, except both arms can be held out to the side, palms forward, or in front of the chest, like a prayer. Come back up by pushing forward off the back foot into the initial position. Change feet with a ginga, until in fig. 3 (No. 2) position, and then drop back into the negativa normal (no hands) on the other side.

Repeat until your thighs are burning.

Pointers

At no point do your hands touch the floor. In the negativa, you can remain on the ball of the squatting foot, or lower the heel and be on the flat foot in the negativa. Be aware that if you choose to flatten your foot (as in No. 5), there is more exertion in rising up again. In negativa, the heel of your extended leg can balance on the floor, with the toes pointing up.

✴

Advanced Sequences and Conditioning

72. (A) Bananeira Walking

■ (NOS. 41/42/43)

Do ginga and drop to cocorinha, put both hands on the ground and stand up into a bananeira, walk backward and forward on your hands for as long as you can, and drop to a ground movement.

Pointers

Work alone or opposite a partner. Look through your arms to the front in bananeira.

✦

73. (A) Bananeira—Cabeça no Chão (Bananeira Push-Ups)

■ (NOS. 40, 41)

Go into a headstand. Push up into a handstand. Slowly lower yourself into a headstand again. Repeat as many times as you can.

Pointers

For extra balance training, try to do a series of these without putting your feet on the floor. This will build a lot of strength and improve your balance for all your upside-down movements. Don't jerk the legs up to help you push into the handstand.

✦

74. (A) Aú Cabeça no Chão Push-Ups

■ (NOS. 16, 34)

Start an aú, slow and controlled, bending your arms so that the top of your head touches the ground; push up and continue the aú to completion.

Pointers

The difference between this and a regular aú cabeça no chão is that instead of having one foot down when you touch your head on the floor, and the other foot down when you raise your head again (as in movement No. 34), here you will lower and raise your head during the course of the aú without putting either foot down. Do not cannon yourself head first at the floor like a missile, but lower and raise your body using the muscles of your arms, shoulders, and back to control the movement.

✷

75. (A) Gato Strength Training

To increase strength for your gato, kick up into a handstand against a wall, with your fingertips quite close to the wall. Holding this position, shrug and lower slowly while remaining in the handstand position the whole time.

Pointers

When you shrug, breathe deeply and concentrate on flexing your back, your arms, your abdominal muscles, your thighs, and holding the flex for a few breaths before releasing the back into the regular handstand. This is an exercise favored by gymnasts training strength for the back handspring (gato in capoeira).

✷

76. (A) Pião de Cabeça into Bananeira

■ (NOS. 63, 41)

Turn a head spin and control yourself to a stop, facing a partner or a predetermined focus point. From this position, preferably without putting a foot on the floor, press up into bananeira.

Pointers

Begin by trying one turn and then the press. Begin and end the head spin facing in the same direction. To add difficulty, do more spins and once you have pressed up into the bananeira take a few steps forward and backward on your hands.

◉

77. (A) Aú Batendo (Scissor Kicks)

■ (NO. 47)

Either working on a partner's hand or kicking into mid-air, hit an aú batendo, one leg to the front, one back, then swap legs with a robust chop, and repeat as many times as you can, kicking left foot–right foot–left foot–right foot, while remaining in the upside-down position.

Pointers

Make sure that your arms are wide and your fingers splayed. Look to the front directly through the middle of your arms with your weight centered equally between the two hands before you begin the scissoring movement. If you do it fast, with both legs working at the same speed, so they change and counterbalance each other equally, you can find a rhythm and repeat this many times before losing balance.

◉

78. (A) Player 1: Bênção
Player 2: Esquiva—Ponte—Walkover

■ (NOS. 83, 91)

Player 1 does a bênção and Player 2 leans back in the esquiva. Player 2 brings his two arms up straight above and beyond his head and leans back, falling into a ponte and walking over.

Pointers

Make sure you really do the esquiva—do it so you mean it—to avoid the incoming kick. Immediately take your two hands in front of your chest, palms together, and then straighten out your arms. With your feet shoulder width, bend back. It is vital to powerfully flex the muscles at the back of your thighs and your buttocks to gain the solid base to fall into the ponte.

Focusing on your hands, and keeping the arms locked out straight, bring the hands to the ground. Your feet remain in the same place and you continue clenching the buttocks as you do that back bend. As with gato, do not bend the arms or you will bang your head. Look at your hands throughout.

From the ponte, walkover as described in movement No. 91.

❄

79. Tesoura Jumps

■ (NOS. 95/96)

Player 1 slides toward Player 2 in tesoura (see Nos. 95/96). Instead of escaping in an aú as we have seen, this time Player 2 will leap forward over the head of Player 1 into a tesoura position of his own and begin sliding back. Player 1 bounces up into cocorinha and dives over Player 2 into tesoura position and begins sliding back; Player

2 bounces up into cocorinha and dives over Player 1 and begins slid-ing back. They repeat this, alternating as many times as they can manage while retaining good form.

Pointers

The first thing to be sure of is to leap parallel to the ground, but far enough that you clear the head of the player doing tesoura. If you land on their head with your leap forward you will probably hurt them at least a little bit, if not a lot. If you were watching this from the side you would see a constantly moving tesoura, one sliding, one leaping the whole time.

Note: When you leap into tesoura, keep your feet as low as you can manage. You should not leap into bananeira and then drop into tesoura; you should already almost be in tesoura position when your hands hit the ground, and then the feet drop a second later and you immediately begin the slide back. This is a popular sequence in capoeira shows.

❂

80. Meia Lua de Compasso— Pião de Mão

◼ (TWO PLAYERS) (NOS. 32, 64)

Player 1 does a meia lua de compasso to Player 2. Player 2 kicks up into a pião de mão directly following the meia lua.

Pointers

Player 1: Be aware that as Player 2 kicks up for the hand spin you are particularly vulnerable to getting kicked directly in the face if you bring your head forward. Remember that to start a hand spin, you need to cross a hand in front of your body, say your right hand, and as you kick up your left leg, you exchange hands, crossing them over each other to create the spin. Just try for a single 360° turn to begin with, and don't expect to be a spinning top first try. At the same time, don't be too satisfied with something that looks so like aú normal that it in fact *is* aú normal.

❋

81. Espinha Forward and Reverse

■ (NO. 68)

Espinha forward, and without turning around or changing direction, espinha straight back again in reverse.

Pointers

Everything will be literally in reverse order. Look at the photos in movement No. 68 in reverse order to see what is happening for this sequence. Remember to always train both sides of your body, so once you've done it forward and reverse one way, turn around and do it the other way.

❋

82. Espinha Wheel

■ (NO. 68)

Here you do a frontal espinha in the same spot, and when you land, you espinha again (in the same spot). On landing, bring the leg back and take off again for a third one in the same spot. Just keep turning over like a wheel.

Pointers

If you lead off with your right foot to the front, you will land on your right foot, so when your left foot comes down sweep it straight through to the back and begin immediately to tip forward for the next espinha. Do three or more in one direction, then turn and do three more leading off from the other foot.

❋

83. Queixada—Espinha

◼ (TWO PLAYERS) (NOS. 18, 68)

Player 1: Ginga and do queixada either to north, south, east, or west (you can vary it). Player 2: Duck under the queixada with the beginning of your espinha and follow through to completion after the kick has passed over you.

Pointers

Player 1: Queixada slowly and calmly (devagar). Give Player 2 time to practice coordinating the aú espinha meshed in with the queixada.

❋

84. Armada—Meia Lua de Compasso sem Mão (Chibata): No Foot Down

◼ (NOS. 19, 50)

A very fast and powerful combination of two kicks without returning the kicking leg to the ground between them.

Pointers

To practice this you might begin by warming up with regular armada and chibata, returning the kicking foot to the ground between them. Then move on to the no-foot-down version. After armada has passed its apex, swing your head downward at the ground to propel your chibata leg up and around. The swing-down of the head must begin as soon as the original armada has passed its halfway point.

❋

85. Bananeira—Queda de Rins Push-Ups

■ (NOS. 38, 41)

This is an advanced push-up. Begin in a bananeira and slowly drop into a queda de rins, with your two feet and head off the floor, resting the weight of your torso with your waist on one elbow. From this position, push up into bananeira again, and do the same thing on the other side. Unlike the queda de rins in No. 38, the hips will be facing more front-forward so that the feet can be held off the ground and the torso balanced on the elbow, ready for the push-up.

Pointers

To build strength for this it is worth beginning with bananeira push-ups. Start in a regular bananeira and practice slowly lowering your head to the ground. If you can't push up again, no problem. Practice starting in the bananeira and lower. This "negative rep" will build strength.

If you are a beginner at this, you can do the bananeira with your feet against a wall and slowly lower yourself onto the top of your head. Keep your body under control so you don't bang your head. Once you have developed sufficient strength to lower and rise in and out of bananeira at least 10 times with strength to spare, you can try bending your head to the side in the down position and lowering even further until your waist tucks on the elbow. Then push up.

Some handstand specialists do these with their hands on two chairs (feet can be against a wall), and the head lowering down in the middle, then pushing up. This allows the player to handstand through a greater range of movement than a regular handstand push-up and would approximate the strength needed for a bananeira— queda de rins push-up.

Note: Don't try this last exercise until you can do regular bananeira push-ups for 15 to 20 repetitions. It may take a few months, even a year, of regular three-times-a-week specific training at the bananeira push-up to get to that stage, so don't worry if you can't do even one rep to start with.

❂

86. Bananeira—Lower into Cabeça no Chão, into Escorpião Cabeça no Chão

■ (NOS. 41, 40, 66)

Once you have built some serious upper-body strength with bananeira push-ups, might as well put it to good use with impressive combinations. Aú slowly into a bananeira and hold the position. With control, lower yourself to bananeira cabeça no chão, and then equally slowly take your legs back into a perfect escorpião.

Pointers

Having done the sequence above, you can reverse this and bring your feet back into regular bananeira cabeça no chão and push up into bananeira and aú out again to finish the sequence. If you can do this, you probably won't need to be told to keep breathing.

❂

Miscellaneous Exercises

87. Ginga

■ (NOS. 1, 2)

Ginga opposite a partner or with a cavalete. Play different kinds of music—traditional Angola, classic Regional, and faster, more contemporary capoeira music. A CD is good, or if you know capoeiristas who will play music for this exercise and vary the tempo, so much the better. Only ginga and really get into it. Feel how different kinds of berimbau music and different styles or songs affect your own rhythm as you ginga. Sometimes it is good to do this in total darkness, so it is just you, the ginga, and the music.

Pointers

Play only capoeira music that you like, even though it is varied.

❖

88. Mirroring

Ginga opposite your partner and watch them very closely. Copy everything that they do. If they wipe their nose, you copy it. They lunge with the weight on their left leg, you lunge with the weight on your right. Then they begin to play. Do the same as they play, copying every move as if you are playing your own reflection in a mirror.

Pointers

Breaking the usual training principle of playing close to your partner, you might want to distance yourself a bit more in this exercise so that you don't need to esquiva to avoid the other player's kicks.

❖

89. Focusing

Play a partner and resolve to watch them like a hawk throughout the game (you don't have to look into their eyes). But wherever you are in the roda, and whatever technique you do, don't let your gaze stray from your partner's movements for even a fraction of a second.

Pointers

Beginners should be careful not to turn away from the opponent when doing rolé. If you tuck your chin in as you turn, and concentrate on turning the head first before kicking, there is never any need to stop watching your opponent.

☀

90. Aú Quebrado

■ (NO. 46)

Opposite another player or opposite a cavalete, aú quebrado east, come back to ginga, (one ginga maximum), and aú quebrado west. To make it more difficult, aú quebrado east, and upon landing back on your feet, immediately aú quebrado west without a ginga in the middle. See how many times you can do it back and forth.

Pointers

Keep the form of your techniques as perfect as you can make it.

☀

91. Bananeira Quiver

■ (NO. 41)

Go into a bananeira, legs in the air and splayed, so your feet are about shoulder width apart. Quiver both your legs rapidly until your whole body shakes and vibrates while remaining in the bananeira position.

Pointers

You can practice the quivering part of this movement standing upright to get the feel for it. Stand with your feet shoulder width apart, on the balls of your feet with your hands outstretched in the air, like a bananeira only upright. Very quickly, with small movements, shake your legs from the knees and thighs until your whole body begins to vibrate rapidly. Stay as relaxed as you can and don't flex your muscles. This is also a good warm-up movement.

✦

92. Stationary Esquiva

Imagining that the balls of your feet are super-glued to the floor, stand in front and within kicking range of a partner. The partner can kick front, turning, and roundhouse in any combination and from any direction. Keeping your feet glued to the same spot 100% of the time, esquiva away from the kicks using only the bend and gyration of your waist and torso. You can fall back into queda de quatro, or down into cocorinha and resistençia, but should not change the position of your feet on the floor.

Pointers

The kicker should work into this slowly. The point of this exercise isn't to send a bênção or chapa battering into the face or solar plexus of the defending player. The purpose is to restrict the movement of the feet in order to increase the player's attention to their waist and upper body during esquiva.

The kicker shouldn't move forward. Stand about the length of your outstretched leg away. No big steps forward so that the defender's position becomes impossible. Defenders should remember that queda de quatro is not a good esquiva from a front kick.

❂

93. Verse-Chorus Breathing with Singing

Two players play, during which one sings the verse of a capoeira song, and one sings the chorus. Keep singing no matter how tired you get.

Pointers

Normally when you are playing in the roda, you will not also answer the chorus, let alone sing the verse. Here, you do. If you don't know any songs, it isn't difficult to find some on the Internet, and it's a simple thing to buy a capoeira CD from an online store. It's best to do this with a short, simple song like a corrido, where you don't require too much brain activity to remember the lyrics.

❂

94. Meia Lua de Compasso— Rabo de Arraia Chasing

■ (TWO PLAYERS) (NOS. 32, 33)

Player 1 aims a meia lua de compasso or rabo de arraia at Player 2. Player 2 drops down onto all fours, two hands and two feet, like a dog or a bear, and walks in toward the outside edge of Player 1's support leg.

Pointers

Drop to all fours immediately when you sense the kick coming. If you keep "animal walking" very close to the outside edge of the kicker's support leg, then the kicking foot can't hit you. If Player 1 then decides to change tactics and kick around for a meia lua de compasso or rabo de arraia in the other direction, he will also have to change support legs, so you simply change direction and stick like glue to the outside edge of the other leg until you figure out what you're going to do next.

✦

95. Queda de Quatro Tag Warm-Up for a Group

■ (NO. 11)

All players in the group fall into queda de quatro, and one or more are chosen as the chaser(s). Also in queda de quatro, the chaser attempts to catch everyone else in the group by touching them. You are all moving around in the queda de quatro position (like spiders).

If caught, the players stand, feet shoulder width apart, and squat up and down into and out of cocorinha repeatedly. They can be saved by a free player leap-frogging over their head (while in the down position of the squat) and then doing a tesoura through their legs (in the up position of the squat). Once saved, they drop into queda de quatro and "spider run" away from the chasers again.

Pointers

When you do the cocorinha squats, don't lean forward in the down position, although you may want to lean a bit when being leap-frogged over. You can also stop squatting when a player is doing tesoura through your legs (so you don't sit on them as they go through). When the chasers have caught everyone in the group (i.e., when everyone is squatting up and down and there is no one left in queda de quatro), the round is over.

Continue until everyone is warmed up.

✴

96. Ginga Back and Forth, and Change Direction

■ (NO. 1)

By bringing the feet alternately forward of the center (center is the position represented by figs. 1 and 3 in movement No. 1) on each changeover in ginga, a player can move forward. By bringing the feet just back of the center on each changeover, the player moves backward. In this exercise, ginga normally, the difference being that the feet return forward or back depending on which direction you want to move.

To turn, when you sweep the ginga foot back, pivot also on the support foot 90° for a quarter turn or 180° for a full change of direction. Do this while maintaining the ginga unbroken.

Pointers

Ginga naturally, practicing turning and moving back and forth. To break up the stepping of a ginga, when the back left foot (for example) returns to center, instead of then bringing the right foot to the back, just bring the left foot back for a second time in a row. There are no hard and fast rules that say the feet need to be brought back and forth alternately each time in ginga. Improvise and experiment with footwork while maintaining the basic structure.

✴

97. Macaco Spinning

In a space where you have some room to maneuver (for example, one end of a gym to another), do a macaco with your left hand beginning the reach back over your head. As soon as this macaco is complete, segue into a second macaco with the right hand reaching back over your head. Repeat left, right, left, right, in a continuous line until you've reached the end of the gym.

Pointers

This is a very effective way to train coordination and the macaco, and will also increase your ability to do this movement spontaneously without a small "rehearsal" or lead-in that telegraphs your intention in advance.

❖

98. Capoeira Solo

Capoeira solos are quite common in batizados and during shows for the general public. They consist of a short sequence performed by a single player, in which they link a series of movements to demonstrate capoeira and show their skill.

Work out a solo consisting of ten or fifteen techniques, lasting approximately a minute or a minute and a half, that you would feel comfortable showing during a demonstration of capoeira.

Pointers

Don't feel you have to do very complicated techniques in a solo. The main thing is that you use techniques you know you have nailed in practice, so you'll be fine doing them in a solo. Keep the quality of the movements at a good standard and link them together smoothly, following the rhythm of whatever music is playing.

❖

99. Magic Berimbau

Ironically, there is no berimbau in this exercise, nor is it magic (yes, I know it's not ironic, but . . .). Children like to do this as a warm-up in the children's class. One person has what they say is a magic berimbau. It's magic because it's invisible.

When the person waves it east, everybody has to esquiva east. When the person waves it west, everyone esquivas west. When the magic berimbau is brought straight down, all must cocorinha with the arms crossed above the head. When the person jabs it forward, all must esquiva back, and when the berimbau makes a circle in the air, all must duck under it as it passes over the top of the circle and aú over it as it sweeps past at the bottom of the circle.

Pointers

Take it easy with the magic berimbau, as it's a lot easier to wave it around than escape from it.

❋

100. Pulo da Onça

I'm leaving this space blank, so you can fill it in yourself. Check the glossary below if you don't know about the pulo da onça. If you have any good ideas for this space, please email them to info@capoeira.no and we'll post them on our website. Thank you. Good training and muito Axé.

❋

100 USEFUL WORDS
AND PHRASES

1. Academia. A capoeira club, school, or academy. Also: *Escolar.*

2. Alto. High, to play high.

3. Aluno/Aluna. Capoeira student.

4. Angoleiro. Someone who plays the Capoeira Angola style.

5. Arrastão. A capoeira technique that grabs both legs and pulls them out by the hem of the trousers

6. Ataque. An attack technique in capoeira.

7. Axé. The power of the Orixás (gods of the Yoruban-Brazilian religion Candomblé), life force, good energy, cosmic vibrations

8. Baixinho. Playing low *(jogo de baixo).*

9. Balão. A capoeira throw. Some were codified by Mestre Bimba in Capoeira Regional.

10. Bamba. A great Capoeira Mestre, a tough guy.

11. Banda. A variety of capoeira techniques to trip an opponent. Vingativa is one example.

12. Bateria. The capoeira orchestra, commonly including a clapperless double bell *(agogô),* a bamboo scraper *(reco reco),* three berimbaus *(berimbau violinha/viola, berimbau medio, berimbau gunga/berra boi),* two tambourines *(pandeiros),* one drum *(atabáque).* In Capoeira Regional: berimbau and two pandeiros.

13. Batizado. A capoeira grading ceremony for rank advancement.

14. **Berimbau.** Main instrument of capoeira, consisting of the *vêrga* or *vara* (the wooden body, made of biriba wood), *cabaça* (the hollow gourd), *arame* (the wire), *vaqueta/baqueta* (a stick to play it with), *moeda/dobrão* (coins or stones to play it with), and *caxixí* (a hand rattle).

15. **Boca de calça.** Pants mouth, cuff.

16. **Brincar.** Childish play, to play.

17. **Calça engomada, não toca no chão.** Play very low, iron the trousers, don't touch the floor.

18. **Candomblé.** African-Brazilian religion, originally from Benin and Nigeria.

19. **Canto de entrada.** The series of chants that follow a ladainha, sometimes called chulas.

20. **Capoeira Angola.** A traditional capoeira style played in Salvador, Bahia, in the early twentieth century. This capoeira was codified and taught by Mestre Pastinha after he and others established the Centro Esportivo de Capoeira Angola in 1941.

21. **Capoeira Contemporâneo.** A term sometimes used to describe contemporary capoeira

22. **Capoeira Regional.** The capoeira style and teaching method founded by Mestre Bimba in Salvador in the late 1920s. He officially opened the first Capoeira Academy, the Centro de Cultura Física Regional, in 1937.

23. **Capoeirista.** One who does capoeira

24. **Cavalete.** A wooden rack or stand to practice capoeira techniques on or over.

25. **Camará.** Comrade, friend, and fellow capoeirista.

26. **Chamada.** A "call" in Capoeira Angola, the same as passo à dois (sometimes called *passagem*).

27. Chula. The call-and-response songs following a ladainha or litany (sometimes called *louvação*), consisting of praise chants—for example, *Viva meu Deus, Viva Meu Mestre,* etc. Also denotes medium-length chants, longer than corridos.

28. Cintura Desprezada. Literally, "scorned hip"; *balãos* (throws) from Capoeira Regional, including *balão cinturado, balão de lado,* and *gravata cinturada.*

29. Comprar o jogo. Buy the game, go in the roda and "buy" out one player, to play the other.

30. Contragolpes. Counterattacks.

31. Contramestre. The player who is an apprentice Mestre, beyond a formado and who may take on many of the responsibilities of a Mestre.

32. Cordão. A belt awarded at a batizado and worn by many capoeira players of Capoeira Regional and Capoeira Contemporâneo.

33. Corpo aberto. An open body.

34. Corpo fechado. A closed body. Can also mean immunity to physical attack, including knives and bullets.

35. Corridos. Short songs of one or two lines sung as call-and-response chants between the main singer and chorus. These are not the same as the chulas sometimes called canto de entrada.

36. Cotovelhada. A strike with the elbow.

37. Cruz. A technique unbalancing the opponent by crossing under a high front kick (bênção for example), catching it on the shoulder, and standing up.

38. Cutelo. A back-fisted hand strike.

39. Dá volta ao mundo. Literally, "to turn around the world." To walk around the inside of the roda in a circle.

40. **Dedeira.** A finger jab to the opponent's eyes.

41. **Defesa.** Defense movement in capoeira.

42. **Desequilibrantes.** Capoeira techniques that unbalance the other player

43. **Devagar.** Slowly, calmly, steady, take it easy! A common exhortation in capoeira rodas.

44. **Discípulo.** Capoeira student. One who follows a capoeira mestre.

45. **Entrada.** Entrance.

46. **Esconder seu jogo.** To hide or disguise the game.

47. **Esquiva.** Escape.

48. **Falsidade.** Trickery, falsity, deceit; an aspect of malícia.

49. **Floreios.** Flourishes; showy capoeira moves.

50. **Formado/Formada.** A "formed" capoeira student. The formado has already been through the stages of *Iniciante* and *Aspirante,* which together take approximately five to seven years.

51. **Frente.** Front

52. **Fuga.** Literally, "flight." Escape techniques.

53. **Fundamentos.** The fundamentals of capoeira: physical, musical, and philosophical.

54. **Galo canto.** The rooster sings, denoting that it's time to begin the roda.

55. **Giro de cintura.** Rotation of the waist.

56. **Godeme.** A fist strike in Regional.

57. **Golpe.** An attack technique, strike, or blow. *Golpe de luta* is a fighting attack.

58. **Golpe de vista.** Seeing the big picture. Perceiving a situation from all angles.

59. **Golpes mortais.** Capoeira techniques that can kill.

60. **Grupo.** A capoeira group.

61. **Guardas.** Defensive positions.

62. **Jeito.** Skill.

63. **Jogador.** Game player.

64. **Jogo.** Game. Often spelled *jôgo*.

65. **Jogo bonito.** Play a beautiful game.

66. **Jogo de dentro.** Inside game.

67. **Jogo de fora.** Outside game.

68. **Ladainha.** Lament, prayer, litany. The long song at the beginning of capoeira rodas, or sung before corridos in Capoeira Angola.

69. **Ligeiro.** Fast

70. **Luta.** Fight

71. **Malandragem.** Deceitful acts involving *falsidade*. The malandro life or values.

72. **Malandro.** A streetwise con-man, tough guy, romantic rogue archetype of Brazilian culture.

73. **Malícia.** A way of thinking and living that involves trickery, cunning, charm, *falsidade*, and an element of practical amorality.

74. **Mandinga.** Can be a synonym for playing capoeira with skill and great cunning.

75. **Mandingueiro.** A capoeira player who has mandinga.

76. **Mestre/Mestra.** A capoeira "master." Specifically one who has "mastered" the art. Different from "slave master," which in Brazil was always *senhor,* not *mestre.*

77. **Miudinho.** Small. To play small, jogo de dentro, a style of Contemporary Capoeira influenced by Capoeira Angola.

78. **Mortais.** Mortal, or deadly. *Golpes mortais* are capoeira techniques that can cause sufficient physical trauma to kill, such as ponteira or martelo.

79. **Movimentos.** Movements.

80. **Ngolo.** The "Zebra Dance," a type of acrobatic combat dance in Angola that took place during the *Efundula* ceremonies of girls who had come of age. Young men would dance the ngolo to win the right to choose a bride. The ngolo is said by many Angoleiros to be the original root of capoeira.

81. **Nome da guerra.** Literally "war name," the nickname often given to capoeiristas at a batizado or within their academy or group.

82. **Palma.** Hand clapping.

83. **Passada.** Capoeira footwork.

84. **Passo à dois.** Stepping in unison. See "Chamada." Ritualized movements played in Capoeira Angola.

85. **Pé da Cruz.** Literally, "Foot of the Cross." The area directly in front of the berimbau where players often wait before entering the roda.

86. **Pião.** Spin.

87. **Pisão.** "Big step" into a side kick.

88. **Pulado.** Jumping.

89. **Pulo da onça.** Literally, "the cat's leap." Named after a Brazilian proverb in which a cat is said to have taught a jaguar every movement it knows, except one. This secret technique it saves to have something left in reserve when the jaguar tries to eat the teacher.

90. **Quadra.** A four-verse call-and-response song type in capoeira, characteristic of Capoeira Regional.

91. **Quebra.** To smash or break.

92. **Roda.** The capoeira circle.

93. **Saída.** Exit.

94. **Seqüência.** Sequence.

95. **Toque.** Rhythm, including berimbau rhythm. Some well-known rhythms include Angola, São Bento Grande, São Bento Pequeno, and Iúna.

96. **Trás.** Behind, back.

97. **Traumatizantes.** Capoeira techniques that may cause physical damage to an opponent's body.

98. **Vadiacão.** Another name for capoeira. Idling around (from the verb *vadiar:* to be idle).

99. **Valente.** Brave. A brave player.

100. **Visão de jogo.** Ability to anticipate what will happen in a capoeira game and to influence events by laying traps.

❂

SOME COMMONLY ASKED QUESTIONS IN CAPOEIRA

How long does it take to get good at capoeira?

Surprisingly, this question gets asked a lot. The easy answer is "How long is a piece of string?" but that's also an unhelpful answer. Some people get "good"—meaning they sing well, play strong berimbau, have a game with plenty of style and variation, even strategy—after three or four years. Those are usually the people who train a lot and dedicate themselves to improving.

It is possible to play a "good" game—meaning one that you enjoy and provides a lot of satisfaction—after a matter of months. In many capoeira schools it takes around seven years to become "formed," that is recognized as a *formado*. It may take an already very good player twenty years or longer to become a *mestre*.

For many people, their criteria of what constitutes "good" changes the better they get. I've talked to people who decide that they have to go back to the drawing board after twenty years, and others who feel like the crowned emperor of planet Capoeira after what appears to be hours.

As I said earlier, though, it is useful to see great capoeira players as sources of inspiration, but my advice is to train only to improve yourself and not as an attempt to become someone else.

How can I train with other people when there's no capoeira club or academy in the town where I live?

I'd say travel to another town where there is a capoeira club. It is also possible to get involved in the whole adventure of applying for a work permit for a teacher to come and live and teach in your town. I am serious, this is a possibility, especially as the very absence of capoeira in your town means that such an applicant wouldn't be taking a job that could be filled by somebody else (which is one of the questions immigration authorities are most interested in).

Having said that, be ready for some heavy-hitting administrative duties if you choose that road. Teachers have to support themselves with capoeira, so there need to be some paying students and a space to teach.

The course a lot of people take in this situation is to forge a very loose link with capoeira on holiday or somewhere, and then start up their own small group of enthusiasts with themselves in charge. This may not be the best course of action, as it starts to spread endless meandering networks of poorly developed capoeira.

I have to go back to the original suggestion of traveling to the nearest town or city where capoeira is available. Sometimes doing what you want to do means making those kinds of sacrifices.

There are fifteen Capoeira schools I could go to in my city. How do I know the difference between them? What's the best?

Request to view a class and ask a few questions to some of the students. It's not like spying. After all, if there are ten or fifteen schools in your town, you want to make a good decision and choose the one you feel comfortable with.

Ask who the teacher's mestre is. If the teacher never had a mestre or a teacher, that could be a problem. Also, if the teacher has never lived in the same country as the mestre or teacher he claims to have trained under, it might raise some questions in your mind. If the answer is a list of names as long as your arm, that is also an eyebrow-raiser. Having said that, people do their best, and an honest teacher with good intentions and a friendly group may be just what you want, *even* if they are 75% auto-didactic (self-taught).

The class can and should be well organized with some structure. There is nothing in capoeira that says classes should be chaotic free-for-alls. Watch a roda. If most of the people in it appear angry and overtly violent and aggressive, it may be just a bad day, or it may be that you want to try elsewhere.

A good capoeira school will start classes generally on time. They'll have a logical payment scheme, a reliable teacher, and a bunch of generally contented-looking students. It may not be a big group, and it may not be the cheapest (or most expensive) or have the slickest home page, but it will just have a good feel about it, what people call Axé in Brazil. If you want to do capoeira, you'll get there.

I'm afraid of standing on my hands—does that rule capoeira out for me?

You don't have to stand on your hands to do capoeira. You only have to stand on your hands to do plantanda bananeira. There are dozens of capoeira movements that don't involve handstanding. You will learn to handle your body weight on your hands with your feet still on terra firma in moves like esquiva, rolé, negativa, and so on. What a lot of people do is stay with the moves they can handle and then one day they realize that they are doing things they never believed they could have done a few months earlier.

Is capoeira at the top level connected to a secret religious cult?

If it is then it must be very secret indeed, because asking around, I can't find anyone in capoeira who's ever heard of a top level, let alone any connection to a secret religious cult.

Can I use capoeira to defend myself against attack?

Many sport martial arts are not suitable protection against the kind of ill-intentioned violence people can meet in the streets of any big city. Some capoeira players are very streetwise individuals, and this may be because they have grown up in conditions that have taught them the skills to handle themselves in dangerous environments.

Capoeira does provide an array of potentially devastating kicks, improve general sensory awareness, self-confidence, and an individual's overall posture and bearing, which may make them a less attractive target for the kind of predators who prey on the easiest-looking victim in a crowd. Having said that, a lot of the moves learned in capoeira classes aren't specifically designed for self-defense against a determined attacker.

Advice on this would be to do capoeira for capoeira's sake, and if you want to learn self-defense, look into some of the excellent specialized systems available today that are structured solely for personal safety.

How do you win capoeira? Are there full-contact competitions?

There are capoeira competitions, though they reached their peak of popularity well over twenty years ago and most capoeiristas don't enter them now. There was a period of time when capoeira competitions were full contact, but as this led to knockouts, often very quickly, the rules were changed by the Brazilian Confederation to competition without contact.

The modern era of academy capoeira was in a sense launched by full-contact competitions. Mestre Bimba, the founder of the Regional system, used challenge matches to gain publicity for his Capoeira Regional style. In a series of full-contact bouts in Salvador in the mid 1930s, Mestre Bimba took on anyone who would fight him, and beat everybody who answered the call. The very next year, in 1937, he opened the first official academy in capoeira's history.

In the early years of the twentieth century, it was generally capoeiristas who were the fighting elite in Brazil. Slowly jiu jitsu started to gain precedence, often by a jiu jitsu practitioner having to defeat a capoeira player to gain recognition for that art.

The fact is, capoeira is too varied to make hard and fast statements about how it develops everywhere. Some mestres are more inclined to contact. The debate about what type of contact should take place has gone on at least since the 1920s when Mestre Bimba was occasionally criticized for doing galopante and hand strikes during full-contact capoeira bouts.

Mestres like the late Sinhozinho or the living Grand Master, Artur Emídio, or even more recently the late, great Mestre Liminha were very strong fighters and capoeiristas. (Mestre Liminha was twice Brazilian heavyweight kickboxing champion.) Most capoeira mestres who enter fighting bouts don't use full contact in everyday capoeira rodas and are clearly able to make the distinction.

Mestre Pastinha, the founder of Salvador's most famous Capoeira Angola Academy, was a critic in the 1950s of too much *vale tudo* (everything-goes fighting) if capoeira used full-contact blows. Mestre Pastinha was quite clear about rules of etiquette in the capoeira roda, which were also designed to protect players from injury.

With the profusion of kickboxing, Thai boxing, and free-style clubs offering semi-contact and full-contact martial arts nowadays, capoeira isn't the first port of call if that is what you are after. On the other hand, there is no denying that some capoeiristas like the element of contact. If I were to say how you win in capoeira, it's by continuing to play it and enjoy it (though that is my personal opinion and only offered as such).

Do I need to learn Portuguese to do capoeira?

For years I reassured myself that you don't need to speak Japanese to do judo, or Chinese to play chess, or English to play football. Then again, you don't sing songs in the language of the country of origin in judo, chess, or football. You can certainly play capoeira without Portuguese, but there are many occasions when being able to speak Portuguese would be like receiving a gift from the gods.

How can I learn berimbau?

If you are buying a berimbau, it's a good idea to buy it with somebody who already has one and knows how to play it. Some music shops order berimbaus and don't know much about the product even though they stock it. Berimbaus vary in quality, and you need to make sure the cabaça (amplifying gourd) and verga (body of the berimbau) are well matched. It is impossible to tell just by looking at them; the berimbau must be played to judge its sound quality. Then practice, and get guidance from an experienced berimbau player.

What's the most important thing in learning capoeira?

Find a good mestre or teacher and be patient with them and with yourself.

◉

ABOUT THE AUTHOR AND THE PHOTOGRAPHERS

Gerard Taylor is a writer and capoeira instructor living and working in the city of Oslo, Norway. He began training in the 1980s and in 1996 received the *formado* grade, and in 1998 the instructor grade from Mestre Sylvia Bazzarelli and Mestre Marcos dos Santos of the London School of Capoeira Herança. In 1996, Taylor established the Oslo Capoeira Klubb with another graduate of the London School of Capoeira, Professora Agnes Folkestad. Over the course of the next decade Taylor trained many hundreds of students. In 2006, the Oslo Capoeira Klubb graduated formados of its own, some of whom demonstrate the movements in *Capoeira 100*.

Since the late 1970s Taylor has worked in various fields of journalism and copywriting, including the Foundation for African Arts, and the *Black Voice* newspaper. He has also contributed articles to *Agogô* and *Brazzil* magazines. Taylor is the author of two previous works on capoeira—*Capoeira: The Jogo de Angola from Luanda to Cyberspace*, Volume One, a comprehensive history of pre-twentieth-century capoeira, published by North Atlantic Books in 2005; and *Capoeira Conditioning*, a whole-body training program using exercises from capoeira, published by Blue Snake Books in 2006.

Anders Kjaergaard and **Sue Parkhill** are professional photographers living and working in London, England. In addition to shooting all the photographs in *Capoeira 100*, they illustrated Taylor's two previous books. They are presently completing work for volume two of *Capoeira: The Jogo de Angola from Luanda to Cyber-space*, which will be published in early 2007.

Kjaergaard and Parkhill are both graduates of the Royal College of Art, where they studied photography in the MA program. They both continue to show their own work internationally as well as collaborating on projects such as this one.

❂